Healing The Family
with
BACH FLOWER ESSENCES

Healing The Family
with
BACH FLOWER ESSENCES

Yeo Soo Hwa
M.Sc. (Pharmacy), BFRP

Sunnyvale • CA • USA

Copyright © 2005 Yeo Soo Hwa

This book is intended to offer information that can assist you in your efforts towards physical and mental health, either individually or in cooperation with a healthcare practitioner. The information contained is not meant to be a substitute for proper medical attention and care where warranted.

Published and distributed in USA by Yeo Soo Hwa
1220-152 Tasman Dr, Sunnyvale
CA 94089, USA
shyeo@myexcel.com

For orders in Asia, contact Shila Gephel
Blk 145, #09-14, Simei St 2
Singapore 520145
chang68@gmail.com

Book design by: Soo Hwa & The Print Lodge
Cover design by: Lynn Kong

ISBN 0-9747742-6X

First Edition

Printed by
The Print Lodge
Singapore

Dedicated to all families
seeking and willing
to heal

Contents

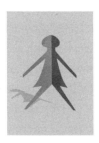

Acknowledgements

Many loving and generous spirits have made this book possible. First and foremost, I want to thank my sister Su Juan and her family – husband Ronnie and their children Shaun and Tara – who kindly hosted and supported me during my visits to Singapore. This book also expresses my appreciation for the people of Singapore who came forward to learn and to work with the essences, and who inspired me with their personal stories and strong desire to be well.

Although it has taken a full three years for the idea to gestate into form, this book was written in record time in October and November of 2003 with great ease and joy. I thank my dear friend Lim Beng Choo for her constant support and feedback during that period, and also for her heroic reminders and efforts to ensure that the manuscript finally turns into print. To my colleague Ann Holmblad in Vermont, I am grateful for her love and presence in my journey, and her review and constructive feedback on the materials presented.

Special thanks go to Lynn Kong and her mother, Soh Lian, for their timely intervention. Mother and daughter put in a formidable effort to create and complete the beautiful cover design in a single day for a total stranger. A small gesture to them but one I will never know how to repay.

It was a wonderful day when I met Matthew Tan from The Print Lodge and interested him in the production of the book. His good heart, professional support, invaluable advice and endless patience were the blessings essential to birth the book in its present form. More than anything else, I cherish the friendship that has sprung from our work together. Heartfelt thanks also go to his designer, Liew Jun Keong for design input and layout of the book, Connie Wai for initial design ideas, and to Clarence Khoo and Patrick Lim for editing and proofreading. If there were an angel taking care of this project, it must be Lim Cheng Cheng who brought to me the necessary individuals to complete this work. Her sweet and loving friendship, wise counsel and dauntless cheer enabled me to cross the finishing line. Equally loving is her husband Chen Hsien who hosted me generously as we saw the end of this project together. To his gentle kindness I am deeply indebted.

My family in America, Willy and Bibi-cat, has been a source of nourishment in every way. Like Einstein, Willy believes that imagination is more important than knowledge. And like a gardener, he tended to me with the utmost patience, loving care and encouragement, allowing me to think and imagine as far as my thoughts can take flight. For this freedom offered so unstintingly, he will always have a special place in my heart. All that I know, all that I have and all that I am today springs from this precious generosity and so this book is as much his contribution as it is mine.

Lastly and most importantly, I give thanks to all the teachers in my life who have led me on this journey of healing and learning. I owe them, as well as my clients and students, an immeasurable gratitude for their inspiration that has turned this book into a reality and for the process that has rekindled some of my own essence.

Yeo Soo Hwa
9 August 2005
Singapore

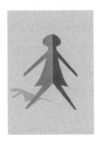

Preface

When asked to write a preface for this book, I was more than delighted to do so. Having known the author since our meeting at the practitioner training of the Bach International Education Program many years ago, I have held the highest regard for Soo Hwa and the knowledge, integrity, clarity and passion with which she shares the work of Dr Edward Bach. Her depth of understanding of Dr Bach and the intricate subtleties of each of the 38 essences is such that I often wonder if the good doctor is somehow standing right behind her as her personal mentor!

In reading over each thoughtfully worded chapter, I am struck by the simplicity and depth of this book. While the book is designed as a beginner's guide to those interested in exploring the Bach Flower Essences for themselves and their families, the material is presented in such a way as to be of interest to those more experienced in the use of the essences, including practitioners. A clear explanation of Dr Bach's theory of healing, concise explanations for each of the essences and the seven groups within which they are categorized along with many pertinent case studies make this book a one of a kind reference for lay persons and professionals alike.

Of particular interest with this book is its focus on those cultures, such as Asian or Scandinavian, for whom the freedom of self-expression is inappropriate and often denied as social and family norms. Soo Hwa points out how the Bach Flower Essences are especially relevant in such cultures, helping to alleviate conflicting feelings within the family by allowing individual members to release and rebalance their emotional distress. In this context, she sheds light on the parent-child relationship, elucidating character traits through essence descriptions, the conflicts that can arise from their interaction, and how to relieve the stresses inherent in each set of dynamics, thereby allowing for the healthier development of both parent and child.

As a teacher and practitioner myself, I highly recommend this book for anyone invested in restoring healthy relationships into their lives. For, in addition to giving an overall perspective on the system of Bach Flower Essences, this book offers insights into the true cause of 'diseased' relationships and true solutions to heal them. It is a hands-on manual that can be of service to anyone willing to take the first step.

Ann Holmblad
Bach Foundation Registered Practitioner
December 2004
Vermont

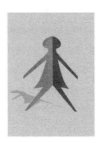

Introduction

My first encounter with Dr Edward Bach was on the pages of his book *Heal Thyself: An Explanation of the Real Cause and Cure of Disease*. His words instantly brought recognition and hope. His views on the inadequate understanding and methods of medical science, on the need to identify and treat actual causes of illness, on the true and spiritual path to health, and on the importance of individuality on that path struck a deep and familiar chord within. The words and ideas mulling in my head for years had finally found form in his writings. This encounter initiated a journey into his philosophy and system of healing that has continued to this day. Over the years, as my understanding of the essences deepen, so has my awe and respect for this man and his knowledge.

This book has been written with the purpose of introducing readers to Dr Edward Bach and his encompassing view on health and healing, and to the Bach Flower Essences as a potent form of self-help family therapy. However, it also contains other subtle but equally important messages that I would like to highlight here. Dr Bach's essential message is that all ills of mankind are spiritual in nature. The etiology of dis-ease – be it mental, emotional or physical – has to be understood where it actually begins or else our desire to conquer it – no matter how brave, how generous and how altruistic – will lead us nowhere.

It all begins with the relationship with ourselves and with the world. By nature, we are all spiritual beings. Spirituality is not the monopoly of religious institutions and persons alone; it is every human being's heritage. Throughout the ages, individuals have experienced this deep and profound longing to return to wholeness. From the saints to the wise sages of old to the plethora of present day gurus teaching ancient and new ways, there has never been a lack of interest in this pursuit. In fact, today, as people over the world begin to understand that external development and materialism cannot assuage this innate yearning, more and more are turning towards spirituality for answers. It can be said, in one way, that everything we attempt in life is the expression of this desire to reconnect with our deepest nature, and all the unhappiness, diseases and suffering of the world a reflection of our failure in this direction.

So where have we gone wrong? We have gone wrong in our ignorance of the true cause of human ills; when we focus on the wrong cause, we necessarily seek wrong solutions. In Chapter III of *Heal Thyself*, Dr Bach said, "The real primary diseases of man are such defects as pride, cruelty, hate, self-love, ignorance, instability and greed ... Such defects as these are the real diseases, and it is a continuation and persistence in such defects after we have reached that stage of development when we know them to be wrong, which precipitates in the body the injurious results which we know as illness." Here he has clearly built us a bridge between our spiritual and physical states of being.

In the tough business of living, many harbor and encourage the belief that spirituality is a luxury and quite separate from life on the material plane. It is quite understandable since no one has taught us that physical health is connected to spiritual health. Besides, we are easily mistaken in our concept of what it means to be spiritual because religious institutions are the only role models available to most of us. Those who do not subscribe to religious tenets are left with no recourse. For those who have given up in this direction, Dr Bach's message is one of hope and urgency. Attending to our spiritual needs is a necessity; for in taking care of our spiritual well-being, we also take care of our physical health. The reverse, however, is not necessarily true and explains relapses in illnesses, a common phenomenon in cancer patients, and why, even in those whose bodies are ravaged by disease to the point of no return, healing is still possible when inner peace and harmony are restored.

Following from this, we can then understand why the true causes of dis-ease are negative personality traits, attitudes and emotions. They are the culprits that fragment our natural wholeness, topple us from equanimity, obscure us with mistaken perceptions, beliefs and habits, and generate inner stress and distress. By falsely identifying with them, we have forgotten and lost connection to our spiritual nature. The ways in which we lose ourselves are both highly individual and universal. Dr Bach used a model of seven group types and 38 essences to describe the pathways in which we have turned away from our essential state. To understand the essences is to understand ourselves and to begin a process of self-discovery, of learning how to recover essence and empower true health in every way.

Making the conscious choice to be true to our spiritual nature is therefore a necessary insurance for good mental, emotional and physical health. However, most of us have not and are not engaged in any form of mental training and therefore would lack the strong mental muscles necessary to effect a purposeful and successful transformation through conscious effort alone. Habitual patterns, be it patterns of thoughts or emotions, take a long time to work on before we become free from their grip. It is important to understand that we are not expected to conquer them simply by will, because there is also an energetic component to this story.

Our negative thoughts – beliefs, perceptions, attitudes – and emotions are energy forms and cannot be eliminated by simply wishing them away. As residual impressions, these energy forms continue to plague us according to their content. Depressing thought, resentment, fear and trauma replay themselves over and over again until these energy forms are worn out or cleared from the system. To purify ourselves of these troublemakers, Dr Bach offered a system of essences that act gently yet powerfully to do just that. Cultivating conscious intent and using the essences to release unwanted energetic forms of past habits in combination is therefore the true pathway to health. It makes the healing complete. It also heralds a message of hope for those who feel condemned, who despair, are ashamed or have given up on themselves. We no longer have to view undesirable traits and habits as our real nature, nor do we have to respond to them with ignorance and negativity. There can be a new view and therefore a new personal reality, which in turn affects the collective reality of the family and society.

This book was first conceived as a public talk called *Bach Flower Essences for the Family* given during a working visit to Singapore in March 2002. The talk was given on three separate occasions to different audiences. The receptivity of minds, the openness of heart and recognition of the truth in this very universal and human system were evident in the audiences. With clients, I found them ready and eager to accept and use them. My experiences touched and impressed upon me the serious need to introduce this topic to a wider audience, and so I was quick to respond to a casual suggestion from my sister to write a book for families.

The contents have been formulated and arranged in such a way as to benefit readers. The sequence of information is important, since each chapter builds on the previous one. It may be tempting to skip to the second half of the book to find immediate answers to a particular problem, but this is discouraged for the following reasons. Because of the unique nature of treating the person, not the problem, one needs to re-orientate one's mind towards this concept before understanding the essences. Besides, an important part of healing is to understand where we are mistaken in our views, beliefs and attitudes, and much of this is discussed in the first half of the book. Many questions that can pop into the mind when reading up the actual application of the essences in healing the family can also be avoided by reading the book in its intended sequence.

There are three main sections and a concluding chapter. *Part 1: Dr Bach and His System* gives the historical background and development of the doctor and the system he discovered. It also presents the basic concepts and principles key to the effective use of the system, and describes the system of 38 essences, what they are and what they do.

Part 2: Understanding Therapy and Usage looks at the unique meaning of therapy in this system, highlights the differences from other healing modalities and reinforces the unique approach of treating the individual's personality to heal rather than focusing effort on the illness or problem. This section also serves to equip readers new to the system with a basic working knowledge of the essences before attempting to use them. It teaches readers how to choose, prepare and use their personal mix of essences, what to expect from their use and advice on how to fine-tune selections and usage to obtain the results they desire.

The second half of the book, *Healing the Family*, is dedicated to specific uses in the family context. It covers four different areas: *Helping Your Family* offers tips on effective helping and how different personality types give or respond to help. *Resolving Family Issues* examines the application of essences to resolve common challenges faced by families. *Growing Up As A Parent* looks at personality traits that generate stress, emotional limitations and conflicts in parents. *Nurturing Your Child* takes readers on a brief journey through the different stages and challenges from birth to young adulthood, and explains how the essences can heal children from their negativity and imbalances and offer them a greater chance to tap into their full potential. Each section is filled with illustrations from case histories drawn from my own experience and practice. Except for open testimonials, clients' anonymity has been respected in every instance by changing and using initials only.

The concluding chapter, *Making Conscious Choices*, discusses the importance of a higher level of self-awareness and conscious decision-making in the family environment, beginning with the decision to bring a child into the world and the meaning of the office of parenthood. Suggestions are offered on how to view and relate to children so parents can bring them up in the most empowering way.

A clear and simple writing style has been adopted to minimize distractions from the essence of the work. Names of essences have been used to describe personality types in an unbalanced state, or a particular negative state or emotion. It is important to understand that there are specific virtues associated with each essence when balance is achieved. For example, the Vine character is domineering, inflexible, bullying when out of resonance.

When they return to harmony, they make the greatest of leaders who act with benevolence and skill. Similarly, the Chicory type, who can be suffocating and possessive in their love, possesses the virtue of unconditional love which becomes apparent when inner balance is restored.

As an Asian and a practitioner, it is my belief that Bach Flower Essences will become an important form of therapy for Asian communities. It is so much in the Asian psyche to be silent and uncommunicative about our genuine thoughts and emotions, and interpersonal dynamics are too enmeshed through generations of tight communal living and influences. It will therefore be difficult for Asians to take to different forms of talk therapies, because the exercise of catharsis, of spewing guts, of 'displaying dirty linen' to another individual is foreign, distasteful and unsafe. This is understandable, and ought to be acknowledged and respected.

Bach Flower Essences, on the other hand, offer Asians the opportunity to work through their negative emotions and attitudes without surrendering long-cherished principles and codes of conduct. The gentle way in which the essences work suits the Asian temperament and its powerful healing properties offer quick relief for conflicts within the intensity of family connections. They can restore lost individuality so essential for creative expression. They can open doors of freedom for many trapped by the cultural habit of stifling and suppressing emotions. Without recourse to relieve the buildup of pressure inside them, loss of control and nervous breakdowns will become increasingly common in the elderly, adults and children. The essences can teach us that there is a place where we can be true to who we are and also be true to those we love. For it is only when we recapture our individual inner peace and harmony that we can live in peace and harmony with our families, society and the world at large. The information in this book can assist families to begin this process of unraveling generations of cultural habits and patterns that are no longer useful in this world we live in.

Change is inevitable and happening at an increasing pace around us. We are required to be resourceful and adaptable in order to flow with external changes, but this is not enough. Those who do not adjust well internally fall behind as outcasts, become maladjusted individuals with psychological illness or frowned upon as social deviants. The essences enable us to adapt emotionally and mentally to change because they help us to keep our center and poise. The resulting inner peace and harmony means we can make the passages of change with less distress and thus maintain our physical and mental health. This is another reason why we need the Bach Flower Essences during these turbulent times.

This book is addressed to all families who are seeking and willing to heal. May this offering become a source of happiness to readers and thanksgiving to Dr Bach for the way he has touched my path. I am deeply indebted to his compassion and dedication to truth. Most of all, I am eternally grateful for the legacy of flower essences that he left behind to empower us to life all over again.

Part I

Dr Edward Bach and His System

In the future, healing will pass from the domain of physical methods of treating the physical body to that of spiritual and mental healing which, by bringing about harmony...will eradicate the very basic cause of disease.

℞
**Dr Edward Bach
Heal Thyself**

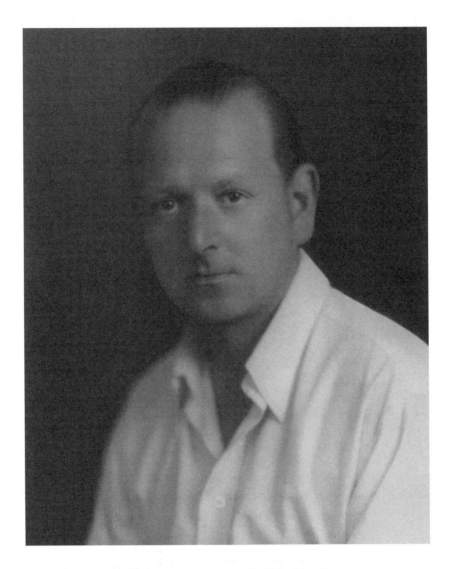

Dr Edward Bach (1886-1936)

M.B.B.S. Bachelor of Medicine and Bachelor of Surgery
M.R.C.S. Member of the Royal College of Surgeons
L.R.C.P. Licentiate of the College of Physicians
D.P.H. Camb. Diploma in Public Health, Cambridge

The Doctor and His Method

The Bach Flower Essences originated in England. They were discovered and developed by Dr Edward Bach, after whom the essences were named. Dr Bach was a well-established physician and medical researcher of his time. He owned a large laboratory where doctors from different parts of Europe would travel to join him in research and to learn from him. He also had a busy consulting practice on Harley Street, where the best of the medical profession of that time were to be found. Through his publications and lectures, he contributed to the advancement of medicine and was regarded as a leading man in his field. You may well wonder why a man of such accomplishment and status in the medical profession would leave behind a legacy of flowers remedies instead. The full story of how this peculiar combination of doctor and flowers developed is narrated by his close assistant, Nora Weeks, in her book *The Medical Discoveries of Dr Edward Bach*[1]. For the purpose of this book, a brief account is given here to provide a historical background for the development of the Bach system of flower essences.

The Early Years

As a child, Dr Bach had a clear knowledge of his direction in life. He possessed an overwhelming sensitivity and compassion for the suffering of fellow living beings, which became the compelling force behind his desire to find a cure for all those in sickness and in pain. Even as a boy in school, he was convinced that he would one day find a form of healing that would cure all diseases and the body, mind and soul, and so he determined to become a doctor. He was a child characterized by an unusual certainty and intensity of purpose, as well as an independent spirit of such strength that no influence, distraction or objection would deter him from his own mind; traits that were to serve him well in the years to follow.

Unwaveringly, he devoted himself to a life in medicine, consciously charting a course that took him from the hospital wards to the fields of Wales, seeking a cure for all ills. Although the major part of his life was dedicated to learning and discovering all he could in medical science, several aspects of it eventually steered him away. During his years of medical practice, he found himself increasingly dissatisfied with the limitations of conventional medicine, which has its focus on treating symptoms instead of addressing the actual cause of disease and curing it. So much of his life's work was therefore geared towards finding a form of healing that directly treats the cause and therefore cures. At the same time, it had to be pure – pure in the sense that it was safe, simple and natural.

He was similarly dissatisfied with the techniques of diagnosis, methods of intervention and substances used to treat patients. The waiting time for test results to confirm a diagnosis can be long, during which nothing much can be done for the patient. Methods of direct physical intervention can cause pain and even injury, further compounding suffering. Substances used to effect a relief are often harmful themselves and thus pose a threat to the patient's already impaired health.

His intuitive and sensitive nature made him a keen and careful observer of human beings. Even as a medical student, his faith in finding a healing solution was not in the theoretical knowledge of books but in careful observation of each individual's unique response to illness. He felt that "the true study of disease lay in watching every patient, observing the way in which each one was affected by his complaint, and seeing how these different reactions influenced the course, severity and duration of the disease." Throughout his life, he was to maintain this practical and empirical approach in his work.

Through his observations, he arrived at a few truths that became the cornerstones for his new system of medicine years later. He became acutely aware of how a patient's personality and emotions have a profound impact on their mental and physical well-being, how it affects their response to their illness and how it affects their recovery from illness. He noticed that the same treatment did not always cure the same disease in all patients. Patients with similar personality traits would often respond to the same remedy, whereas those of a different temperament were helped by other treatment, although they were all suffering from the same complaint. Early on in his medical career, he concluded that the personality of the patient plays a greater role than the body in illness, and therefore must be taken into account in treatment.

We must remember that this was in the early 1900s, an era when such an assertion was contrary to the prevailing view in medicine. The view then, as is now, is primarily a biomechanistic one. In this model, the heart is seen as a mechanical pump; the skeleton a system of pulleys and levers to allow movement; the lungs a pair of bellows for gaseous exchange, and so on. Medical science was and still is powerfully reductionistic, reducing a patient to physical components of the body and designing relief for those parts alone without acknowledging the exquisite uniqueness and totality of an individual.

Dr Bach was therefore a physician well ahead of his times when he decided to seriously explore this connection between emotions, mental states, personalities and physical health. Through his diligent work on the Bach nosodes – oral bacterial vaccines that became the subject of several publications and subsequent fame – and his contact with homeopathy, his convictions grew increasingly strong. Until finally, in 1930, at the height of his career in London, he decided to completely abandon his work there and left for the fields he so loved, penniless but with a mind fresh and determined to start a different journey to discover a new form of medicine.

Dr Bach was to spend the rest of his life trudging the fields and countryside of Wales and England, seeking and finally finding what he was looking for. This period coincided with a quickening of his spiritual growth and an expansion of his intuitive capacities. His senses became so heightened that he could directly experience the healing energy of the flowers he discovered. And so, rapidly, he found them one by one in this fashion. Later on, before each flower that was revealed to him, he was to suffer the mental and emotional state that it treated, sometimes so acutely that he was taken ill. The last 19 of the 38 remedies were discovered in quick succession in this manner over a short span of six months. This process took a toll on the kind doctor's body and is a true testimony to his compassionate spirit, for he suffered much to find the essences he left behind. In the last two years of his life, he settled down at Mount Vernon, now The Edward Bach Centre, and displayed great courage by treating all his patients, no matter how serious their conditions, solely with the essences and effected many astonishing cures.

The elements of this setting were conducive for demonstrating the full power and efficacy of the essences. As a medical doctor, Dr Bach commanded faith and confidence from his patients who came with all types of physical ailments. He had the opportunity to use the essences in a medical setting. Because he saw the essences as medicine, he used them as such even for severe cases with the intention to cure. One of the characteristics of this system is that when a person is acutely out of balance, the swing back to balance is equally swift. This was evident in the many case histories documented by Dr Bach and his colleagues, some of which may seem 'miraculous' in nature to those unfamiliar with the workings of this system.

Nowadays, most flower essence practitioners are non-medical individuals who are not presented with the same opportunity to work with a large number of severely ill patients and to demonstrate as readily the full efficacy of the essences. It is not that they are less capable, just that their status does not deliver the same opportunity. In fact, Dr Bach himself believed that lay people make better users of the essences because they are less complicated and distracted by medical knowledge and training, and can focus solely on the presenting temperament to identify the right essences. This system is meant to be that simple and 'miracles' are to be expected. Events only appear as miracles to our minds when we do not understand how things work. But once we understand the correct pathway to health, any healing is possible.

Unfortunately since Dr Bach's time, the essences are treated less seriously in their ability to cure. A large part of this is due to fear and ignorance, sometimes even from the very people who are practicing them.

❀ The Legacy Of The Flowers

Since Dr Bach's time, the interest in the link between emotional-mental states and physical health has seen a renaissance in the 1990s, setting off a proliferation of healing modalities in an attempt to understand and affect the mind-body connection. This connection has now been accepted even by the medical establishment as an essential component of therapy. Acknowledging the mind-body connection, however, is not sufficient to heal it. We can see this clearly in a couple of examples. In America, two to three out of four visits to the doctor are stress-related. The doctor can acknowledge and advise that the source of the physical symptom is stress, but would not know what the cause of the stress is or how to eliminate it. The common solution is to help the patient cope with the stress by prescribing some anti-anxiety pills or anti-depressants and recommend a change in lifestyle. This problem can also exist in holistic therapies that do not offer the knowledge or a tangible way of working directly on the mind-body connection. In such instances, one is at best engaged in a blind exercise of trying to effect change without really knowing the pathway to bring about the desired change. Sometimes one is lucky and successful, at other times not so.

Dr Bach took us one step further in this direction by establishing a system of essences that are directly related to specific human mental and emotional states. This correlation allows us to use the essences with accuracy of intention and effectiveness to eliminate specific internal events that are creating emotional and physical distress. With a direct pathway and knowledge, it is easy to address the underlying emotions and mental states that are threatening our health, thus making healing fully possible. Such a contribution is revolutionary even by today's standards. Before his death in 1936, Dr Bach stipulated that his system was complete. Used individually or in combination of up to six or seven essences, there are as many as 293 million possible permutations, sufficient to take care of the full spectrum of emotional and mental states that an individual experiences over a lifetime.

Conventional medicine has not made it easy for us to understand our illness nor the medications we use. Medical terminology becomes more and more complex, with many new labels added to describe baskets of symptoms no one understands or knows how to treat. Pharmaceutical companies deliver us new drugs that are slight mutants of each other or old ones repackaged in new delivery forms under new names. The list grows longer by the day and with it, the confusion and disarray of information.

By comparison, the Bach system is attractive in its simplicity; a simplicity derived by turning our attention away from the multitudes of physical expression of dis-ease to the essential cause, the source from where it begins – the person. The direct use of the essences to treat human nature is unique because it deals with the common denominator in all challenges and circumstances of life – the individual who is the *experiencer* of events, whether it be illness, problems in relationships, at work, with life or with death. The fact that all of us respond differently to the same situation indicates that, as individuals, we contribute to the interpretation and response to an event. The number of possible interpretations and responses is as vast as the human race. By returning the common denominator – the person – to balance, every relationship with that center is also healed in a single stroke. From this balanced center, the individual is then able to deal constructively and effectively with the circumstances placed on his or her path.

Another of Dr Bach's contributions is his presentation of the seven basic types of human responses to life. This insight came to him serendipitously at a dinner party in 1928, the same year that saw the birth of his new work.

While observing the dinner guests to pass his time, he suddenly realized that the whole of humanity could be divided into groups of types. As the night continued, he observed everyone in the dining hall – the way they spoke, smiled, moved, ate – and by the time dinner was over, he had worked out his group theory. He came to see how humankind could be classified into seven types according to their predominant response and sensitivity: fear, uncertainty, insufficient interest in present circumstances, loneliness, over-sensitivity to influences and ideas, despondency or despair, and overcaring for the welfare of others.

This presentation of the group theory is itself a therapeutic tool that can initiate a learning process for us to grow in self-knowledge. Self-knowledge plays a crucial role in healing. The essences clear away obscurations, allowing us to understand our individual make-up. What makes me tick as a person? What makes me sad, angry, resentful, or fearful? Where am I most sensitive and vulnerable to stress? What are the habitual perceptions and attitudes controlling my responses? So much of our suffering comes from ignorance and confusion about ourselves, transferred onto our relationships with others and life. We have to check if and where there are errors in the way we have programmed ourselves, for these habitual tendencies dictate our reality. The body is only the hardware that reflects the errors in programming. By knowing where we have erred in our perception, we can correct and even prevent the arising of mistaken perceptions and their accompanying negative emotions that disturb inner peace. Such understanding is wisdom that seals the healing; we heal as we grow in self-knowledge.

✿ In Harmony With True Nature

Dr Bach's philosophy of healing is based on the innate perfection and spiritual nature of living beings. He taught that the cause of disease is a conflict of an emotional and spiritual nature deep within the individual due to "a dissociation between the Personality and Soul." By *Personality,* he meant the way we present and deliver ourselves to the world; a self-image crafted consciously or unconsciously. By *Soul*, he was referring to our true nature, a deep spiritual essence unique to each one of us.

When there is a divergence between who we really are and how we perceive and present ourselves to the world, we suffer from an internal conflict moment to moment. As long as this conflict is not acknowledged and corrected, it reverberates within us for days, months and years and in many cases, for life. The disharmony expresses itself in different ways, first emotionally and mentally generating internal stress. Left unattended over long periods of time, this ongoing dissonance begins to interfere with the normal functioning of the physical body and physical symptoms start to appear. What most of us call illness or disease is the product of a much longer-term condition. Dr Bach himself called disease "a consolidation of mental attitudes". It is as if a negative emotion or mental state has become encrusted in the body. To return to health, we need to restore our natural state. We do this by using the essences to eliminate distorted perceptions, negative attitudes and emotions that obstruct our true nature and its expression. Consciously, we also need to make consistent efforts to empower ourselves in the opposite direction even as we release these unconscious programs that run our lives. True health comes when we are in harmony with our true nature.

The word 'disease' is commonly used to describe a physical ailment, but when we use it according to its original intent – *dis-ease* – then we can understand how its broader meaning embraces any state of a person ill at ease or not at ease with him or herself. In this system of healing, emotional dis-ease and mental dis-ease are the illnesses we need to focus our attention on. They are the precursors and underlying cause of physical symptoms and so, in every case of using the essences to help someone, we have to keep returning to the original cause and treat it accordingly. This then is the basis on which Dr Bach approached healing.

Here a word of caution ought to be inserted in case readers have concluded that the author is advocating the Bach Flower Essences as the one and only true method to be adopted for all conditions. It is true that the essences are relevant in all conditions. However, we should not simply take them and ignore the bleeding or the ulcer or the pain in the body. We have to take care of that as in every medical treatment. The point to remember is that until we address the underlying mental and emotional cause, complete healing cannot take place. The physical stress is but a symptom of a deeper and more essential distress.

All existing systems of healing knowledge are necessary; they make up a spectrum of techniques that can be skillfully applied to specific complaints for specific individuals at specific times. There is no contradiction amongst the different modalities. Healing is an art, the art of finding the right tool for the right patient at the right phase of the healing process. To illustrate this, let us think of someone who has just been hurt in an automobile accident, in severe traumatic stress and losing blood. Conventional medicine is unsurpassable in its techniques for intervention in an emergency like this. The torn artery can be clipped to stop bleeding; blood from a donor can be infused to compensate for excessive blood loss; an electric shock can be applied to revive heart muscles and so on. There is no time to slave over a pot of herbs while the patient is dying on the table. Indeed, using the wrong method for the wrong situation may even cost a life! Conversely, conventional medicine has failed miserably in many chronic and especially emotionally-induced illnesses. Patients are put on years of treatment, spend a fortune on medications, and suffer on without hope of a full recovery.

Each modality has its role in the different phases of the healing process. To identify the right modality, we need to ask questions: Are we treating at the causal or resultant state? The acute or the chronic? Except in those instances where immediate and aggressive intervention is required, we are still much ruled by our individuality. Just as we take to different foods, so our likes and dislikes predispose us to different practitioners and different techniques. When we work with a healing practitioner and method that we feel comfortable with, we are more likely to co-operate and respond. This element of individual affinities plays a far greater role than most want to or can recognize, but still it has to be respected and honored. It does not mean that if a technique has not worked for us, then it must be useless. Neither does it mean that if a technique works for us, then it is the best. What works and does not work is only applicable in the context of the individual. Until we come to this understanding, we continue to hold biased, exclusive, fragmented and incomplete views of the place for each healing modality. When practitioners are incomplete in their understanding, their patients also fall prey to their incomplete views and ignorance is propagated.

Thus far, Dr Bach has made us aware of the potency and toxicity of our negative perceptions, attitudes and emotions. They are not the harmless irritants and innocent nuisances of life as we tend to view them. Our personality, habitual attitudes and emotions impact every aspect of our lives; they are the very cause of problems in our family, relationships, spiritual practice and work. They determine whether we accomplish our goals and dreams, have a fulfilling life or not, and our overall psychological and physical health. Sound healthcare needs to begin by paying attention to our internal states of mind and emotion. Heeding these important signals and taking care of them promptly, we can avoid much of the pain and suffering that comes when we are struck down by a full-blown physical illness.

Unlike the fluctuating stock market, fashion trends, technological advances that change at a dazzling speed, and the overwhelming array of diseases that appear with new names and new drugs, human nature throughout the ages and everywhere in the world remains essentially the same. People still fear and hate, get impatient and resentful, lose confidence and hope just as they have since time immemorial. The ignorance and hatred that fuelled the Crusades in the Middle Ages are no different from the cause of unrest in the world today. The current fear of AIDS is no different from the fear of tuberculosis or influenza at the turn of the last century. Heartaches and jealousy – the substance of classic love tragedies – still play themselves out in today's soap operas. Whether it is the 1930s or the present century, all 38 essences remain potent and relevant for healing regardless of race, culture or creed. This system is a medicine that will outlive any external changes in this rapidly changing world of ours. They have a timeless application and that is the reason why Dr Bach called his essences "the medicine of the future".

There is much to be admired of this kind doctor who was never recognized for his greatest contribution to mankind in his lifetime. Throughout his life, he displayed great courage in pursuing his personal calling with a devotion and purpose that is truly admirable. Like so many great masters of the past, truth and compassion were far more important to him than worldly distractions and concerns. Nearly seven decades after his passing, people are only just beginning to appreciate and respect the purity and potency of the flower essences he left behind as a gift for mankind, and for the depth of his understanding of human nature. It is this wisdom in understanding human nature that allows complete healing to take place, for we cannot hope to remedy ourselves or others we do not understand. As long as we fail to understand, we will perceive symptoms to be causes, we will seek answers and cures outside of ourselves, we will continue to absorb incorrect views and inaccurate perceptions as the true nature of things, and react to them with a multitude of disturbing emotions. Identifying the wrong problem, we necessarily seek wrong solutions. Without understanding human nature, we cannot hope to begin the journey of becoming whole again.

Dr Bach provided us with a much-needed compass that points to a new and true pathway to health. He said, "The physician of the future will have two great aims. The first will be to assist the patient to a knowledge of himself ... The second duty ... will be to administer such remedies as will help the physical body to gain strength and assist the mind to become calm, widen its outlook and strive towards perfection ..."[2] Armed with self-knowledge and the essences, we can all become our own healers and help others who are seeking to do the same.

---

[1] The Medical Discoveries of Dr Edward Bach by Nora Weeks. Published by Keats Publishing Inc., 1973.
[2] Heal Thyself: An Explanation of the Real Cause and Cure of Disease by Edward Bach, M.B.B.S., D.P.H. Published by The C.W. Daniel Company Limited, first published 1931, reprinted 1994.

2
The Thirty-Eight Flowers

The Bach system consists of 38 essences specially selected by Dr Bach for their unique properties. They are prepared from the flowers of plants, trees and bushes growing wild in England, with the exception of four. The blue-flowered Cerato is a cultivated plant indigenous to Tibet, China and the Himalayas. Olive and Vine were and still are prepared from olive trees and grapevines that grow well in the warmer Mediterranean regions of Spain, South of France and Italy. One of the flower essences, Rock Water, is an anomaly; it is not even a flower. Dr Bach's source of Rock Water was from a healing spring close to his Mount Vernon home in Sotwell; it was known to have healing properties for the eyes. In later years, this water was taken from a selected well or spring known for its power to heal the sick.

The essences are extracts of the healing energy of the flowers and the single healing water. They are still harvested and prepared in the way pioneered by Dr Bach, under stringent but loving care by the trustees of The Edward Bach Centre. Dr Bach discovered that it was possible to transfer the energy of the flower into water as a medium with the help of the sun's heat. Twenty of the 38 essences are prepared in this manner. Flowers that bloom in the colder seasons, when direct and continuous sunlight for proper potentization is not possible, are boiled instead to extract their essence. The mother tinctures thus prepared are preserved in alcohol and, through a series of dilutions, are transformed into the stock concentrates that are sold in the stores. For those interested in the botanical descriptions of the flowers used and details of these two methods, an excellent reference is *The Bach Flower Remedies: Illustrations and Preparations*[1] written by Nora Weeks and Victor Bullen, close assistants to Dr Bach.

Today there are many commercial lines of flower essences in addition to the Bach system, but they all utilize the same potentization and usage method developed by Dr Bach, and subscribe to a similar philosophy and approach to healing. The major difference is in the type and number of flowers that are used for each system. Dr Bach was particular about the types of flowers that he used. They must be non-poisonous for he was convinced that poisonous substances and plants have no real place in the healing of the human being. He also stipulated that only the healing energy of the flower heads is to be harnessed. In the flower is concentrated the life of the plant, its seed containing the essential life force that has the potential to bring forth an entire new plant. Finally, the flowers must be subjected to minimal processing when extracting their healing powers.

Those who are new to flower essences often confuse them with essential oils in aromatherapy. Essential oils are aromatic substances extracted not only from flowers, but also from different parts of the plant such as roots, seeds, leaves and stems. They have healing properties by virtue of the chemical constituents of the oils, which may possess anti-fungal, anti-viral, antioxidant, anti-bacterial, antiseptic or immune-stimulating properties relevant to physical healing. Although there are some who use the oils for emotional healing, this form of therapy from its time of origin and up till today is used mainly as alternative medicinal agents in an approach that remains largely allopathic. The method of extraction is much more elaborate than the pure transfer of energy. The Bach Flower Essences, however, do not carry any physical or chemical components of the flowers and they address solely the inner disharmonies within a person's consciousness. This is of special benefit to those who are sensitive or allergic to different plant substances.

How The Essences Act

Each of the 38 essences treats a specific negative emotional or mental state. 'Negative' here does not connote a value judgment of good or bad; rather it is used to describe a state that blocks or obscures our true nature and expression. It is described as negative only because it brings about an undesirable result, which could be an experience of fear, frustration, confusion or despair. The flowers contain vibrations that resonate at specific frequencies corresponding to those positive qualities natural to us. When we take the essences, we are essentially re-setting or re-tuning our energetic system to its natural balance and harmony with the help of an external agent, which is the flower vibration corresponding to the specific positive state that has been obscured or blocked in expression. In the process, the vibrations of toxic attitudes and emotions generating mental, emotional and physical distress are flushed out of the energy body. When harmony is reinstated in the energy body, so is balance restored to the physical body.

The goal of therapy, then, has never been to change anything in us. Instead, the essences serve to reconnect us to our natural state. It is in recovering our core essence that we become whole again, for we can only be truly happy when the outer personality is in harmony with our spiritual nature. This harmony and oneness is the cause of good mental and physical health. In Dr Bach's own words, "Treat people for their emotional unhappiness, allow them to be happy, and they will become well."

Many people wonder if they have to be on the essences for life in order to get well. The answer is no. The effectiveness of therapy really depends on (1) a good understanding of how and what the essences do, (2) identifying an accurate selection of essences, (3) consistent usage, and (4) the diligence of the user in reaching his or her desired goal. With these elements in place, it is possible to become totally free of the undesired traits, attitudes and emotions that plague us. Over the years, I have seen my clients move beyond their initial essences to a place where they no longer need them. Things that used to frighten, disappoint or anger them simply cannot and do not have that impact anymore. The reverse is also true. Initially, we may categorically reject an essence, thinking we will never have occasion to use it in our lives. Over time, as layers of the outer façade are peeled away, we could discover that this particular essence trait actually underlies the problems we had before. For those embarking on a spiritual path, the essences are delightful companions on a journey of self-discovery. They show us hidden aspects of ourselves and at the same time heal us from them. It is useful to bear in mind that you can take this form of therapy as far as you want to go and you can also stop it whenever you want. This is a personal choice, even when you are working with a Bach practitioner.

Advantages Of Flower Essence Therapy

The essences can be taken alone or in conjunction with other treatments, allopathic or homeopathic. As such, they act as a very helpful and relevant adjunct therapy to most healing modalities. Because the essences are energy extracts, they do not interact with any physical or chemical substance, so they present no interactive problems with any type of medicine, food and drink. Taking with or without food is of no relevance.

However, the essences are not meant to be a substitute for medical treatment. It is true that physical symptoms can go away when the mental-emotional states are returned to balance. Nevertheless, severe medical conditions do need to be treated by the appropriate professional to alleviate the immediate danger and suffering of the individual. There is no contradiction between taking care of the physical symptoms and taking care of the underlying mental-emotional cause. This way of mixing therapies can only synergistically facilitate complete and rapid healing.

Because the sources and preparation of the essences are so pure, they are non-toxic and have no adverse effects. Because their purpose is to restore internal balance and natural resonance, they are non-addictive. This is a completely safe therapy, a rare phenomenon in today's world of medicine. As a pharmacist by training, I find this safety factor particularly appealing. Pharmacy law regulates and governs the use of pharmaceutical products. The need for this law comes from the fact that every drug, at some concentration, turns into a poison. There are some extremely lethal ones like digoxin for the heart, fatal in minute quantities, and there are others like paracetamol, which requires an intake of 12g or 24 tablets of 500mg to cause substantial bodily harm to an adult. Nonetheless, there is a definite boundary between therapeutic and toxic doses. So much of medicine is already practiced out of fear – the fear of not understanding the disease compounded by the fear of drug toxicity. Just to be able to relieve one component of this fear is a major accomplishment since fear itself obstructs recovery.

The essences are simple to prepare and use. Because of the minute dilutions required, they are an extremely economical form of therapy. Coupled with their safety, it means that you can help yourself and experiment with the essences freely without worry about side effects, toxicity and adverse interactions. Taking the wrong essences can do no harm; there will simply be no effect and this is the worst to be expected in therapy. Experimentation is also a wonderful way to learn about oneself and to understand the essences.

You can use the essences for all ages, from a newborn to the elderly. Each phase of life presents its own set of problems that can be assisted by the essences. Both animals and plants have also benefited from the essences. The skeptical mind may attribute their actions to the placebo effect. The fact that animals, plants and children respond extremely well to the essences demonstrates that they are not mere placebos. We cannot suggest to an animal, plant or child that they are going to get well with the essences. They do not know what they are given and cannot will themselves to wellness. Critics may also view the essences as a primitive form of therapy, relying solely on empirical evidence to document their efficacy. The reverse argument can also be put forward – that current science and technology are not sophisticated enough to develop machines that are able to detect and measure the energetic healing potencies of these flowers. The arguments can go back and forth, but the easiest way to end doubt and skepticism is to try them and discover for oneself.

The Essences In Practice

In the nearly 70 years since Dr Bach introduced the essences, they have been used widely throughout the world by medical and complementary health practitioners and lay people with no medical background. Doctors, psychiatrists, psychotherapists, midwives, dentists, chiropractors, naturopaths, veterinarians have incorporated the essences into their work with patients. They are also popular with practitioners of alternative methods such as massage therapists, Reiki practitioners and other energy healers.

Medical doctors have found that the essences produce a marked improvement in the emotional state of patients, thereby instilling a positive attitude towards recovery. Patients also become more open and receptive to treatment, eliminating resistance to therapy. In fact, out of economic necessity, flower essence therapy is considered part of mainstream medicine in Cuba today.[2] Medical doctors recommend flower essences to their patients alongside their more traditional pharmaceutical drugs.

In the field of behavioral therapy or counseling, the essences offer tangible assistance because they work directly to release the vibrations of negative emotions, perceptions and attitudes, bringing on relief and freedom from them in a way not seen in other forms of therapy.

J. Herbert Fill, M.D., psychiatrist and former New York City Commissioner of Mental Health states, "I use them almost exclusively instead of tranquilizers and psychotropics, and in many cases they alleviate the problem when all else has failed. The Bach Flower Remedies are extremely sophisticated in their alleviation of specific moods, gentle and yet potent in balancing the body's subtle energy fields. Though subtle in their action, the Bach Flower Remedies are not placebos."[3]

Animals have emotions too, and so holistically oriented veterinarians are increasingly interested in this system. One vet reports, "In those cases with a good match between symptoms and remedy, you can have very gratifying and quick results. I've yet to see adverse effects, which is different than other therapies such as herbs, chiropractic and acupuncture – in some of those cases, I have seen animals get worse after treatment."[4] (Burton D. Miller, Riverhead) And from one dentist's experience: "In my dentistry practice, I use Rescue Remedy, which I find phenomenal if I have to use epinephrine in the anesthetic (epinephrine is necessary for deeper surgeries) and the patient has a reaction to the epinephrine. Epinephrine sometimes will cause heart palpitations. You may have heard someone say, 'When I go to the dentist, I get a shot and my heart starts racing.' Essentially, there is nothing that can be done. You just let it go, and in time it will pass. But I find if I give Rescue Remedy when they react, in a matter of seconds, it's gone. I also use Rescue Remedy for anxious patients, and they find it helps."[5] (Mark A. Breiner, D.D.S., Orange, Connecticut)

Over the years, results have been consistent regardless of the field the essences have been applied and there are many case histories documenting their successful use.

❁ Rescue Remedy

In addition to the 38 individual essences, Dr Bach also formulated a composite preparation called Rescue Remedy that serves as an all-purpose remedy for emergency and stressful situations. Rescue Remedy is the world's best-selling natural remedy for stress relief. Most people first encounter the Bach essences by way of Rescue Remedy. It deserves separate attention for several reasons. Firstly, the American Medical Association now recognizes stress as a major contributor of illness. Fifty to 75 percent of doctor visits are stress-related, making the role of Rescue Remedy significant. Secondly, the most dramatic effects are seen with the use of Rescue Remedy because it is used under acute situations. The more unbalanced the system, the more rapid and profound the return to balance. A rubber band stretched taut snaps back quickly when the tension is released, but gently if it is stretched lightly. The same phenomenon applies here.

Flower Essences in Dentistry

Dear Soo Hwa,

I have been using the flower essences actually since your talk, with more frequency and readiness that it is now part of my dental treatment.

Overall, I reach out for the flower essences whenever I detect fear, resistance, phobia and anxiety in the patients receiving dental treatment. Whether they believe or not in the effectiveness of the essences, I inform them of the flower essences I would give them. I either drop the essences directly into the mouths under the tongue or else have them drink the essences in water. Depending on the issues the patients have, different combinations of Bach flowers are given.

In particular, there was one patient who was a dental phobic and had to take a sedative and tranquilizer before he boards the plane or sits in the dental chair. After the use of Rescue Remedy, he uses the flower essences instead of the drugs to alleviate his anxiety about the aforementioned situations.

In times of emergency, I spray the Rescue Remedy in the vicinity of the patient. Almost instantaneously, there is a change in the emotions of the patients with resulting better compliance and ease of treatment procedures carried out. Again, I emphasize that this happens whether the patients believe in the flower essences or not and irrespective of their cultural, racial, religious differences.

Dr Gan Siok Ngoh, D.D.S.
Singapore

- extracted from a letter to author -

Rescue Remedy contains five essences that together help to calm, stabilize and soothe under acute stress that can occur in a car accident, a natural disaster such as an earthquake, the man-made calamities of terrorist attacks or war, a serious fall, emotional setback or panic attacks. When a person experiences a trauma or shock under those circumstances, the entire system goes out of balance. The five essences act in synergy to counteract the mental-emotional states that arise. The shock in a traumatic event is relieved by the essence *Star of Bethlehem*. Under strain, a person's mind starts to give way or there is a fear of it doing so. *Cherry Plum* takes care of the fear of losing control or the actual loss of control. *Impatiens* releases the tension buildup in the body and mind, and *Rock Rose* reduces the panic and terror. A person in shock can also become numb or drift into unconsciousness. *Clematis* helps to ground them in the physical body.

We need not use Rescue Remedy only under severe conditions. It also serves us well for the small daily stresses of living. A child anxious about a visit to the dentist or an upcoming examination experiences stress. Stress levels rise even for adults who have to take a driving test or prepare for a job interview. We can also be stressed by deadlines at work, public speaking or inter-personal conflicts, when we receive shocking news as in a death, diagnosis of an incurable illness, a broken relationship or financial loss. There are many documented cases of the wide range of use and success of this combination essence. Gregory Vlamis pays special tribute to Rescue Remedy with his collection of stories in the book *Bach Flower Remedies to the Rescue*.[3]

Rescue Cream is formulated in an inert vegetable base for topical application. It contains the additional essence Crab Apple for its cleansing properties to facilitate topical healing. It has found itself in varied use for insect bites and stings, hives and rashes, sore and sensitive gums, tooth extraction or teething in infants, chapped lips, contact dermatitis, cuts, diaper rash, hemorrhoids and burns. Midwives use it in child delivery, massage therapists in their massage practice.

A Word About Stress

Stress is a very commonly used term these days; it is one of those words that has found its way into our vocabulary but has not been clearly defined. According to the Taber's Cyclopaedic Medical Dictionary, stress is defined as "*A condition harmful to an organism which results from the inability of the organism to maintain a constant internal environment.*" In short, stress occurs whenever a person is unable to maintain internal balance and harmony. With that imbalance come certain physical and emotional responses. The symptoms vary widely amongst individuals – from insomnia, ulcers, heart palpitations, appetite loss or overeating to mental agitation, depression and anxiety. By itself, stress does not exist as a disease or medical condition. Treating the stress symptoms therefore does not lead us to a permanent solution.

Every time we experience a negative emotion such as anger, fear, jealousy, uncertainty or grief, we tip the internal scale of balance. The system goes under stress immediately; it is just a matter of whether it is low-grade stress or acute stress. These daily doses of mental and emotional stress have an effect on the physical body. Some individuals, who are more sensitive to their inner balance, can detect and heed the signals and take care of them in time. Many have adopted a pattern of numbing their emotions and inner conflicts. For them, it takes the stress to manifest physically before they attend to it.

Rescue Remedy takes care of the immediate symptoms of stress, but it is the entire 38 essences that relieve stress in the long run. Together, they offer an excellent tool for the daily and sound management of stress and therefore of health.

The 38 Flower Essences

The year 1928 was a memorable one for it marked the discovery of the first three essences in the system and the birth of Dr Bach's group theory. He intuited that the whole of humanity consists of seven groups of personality types, and came to understand that "individuals of each group would not suffer from the same kinds of disease, but that all those in any one group would react in the same or nearly the same manner to any type of illness."

The significance of this discovery was translated into Dr Bach's classification of the 38 essences. He placed them into seven distinct categories of responses that arise under duress, illness or when confronted with the daily challenges of living (Figure 1). They also describe how each one of us can be out of balance internally at any time. The seven basic types are:

1. **Fear**

2. **Uncertainty**

3. **Insufficient Interest in Present Circumstances**

4. **Loneliness**

5. **Oversensitivity to Influences and Ideas**

6. **Despondency or Despair**

7. **Overcare for the Welfare of Others**

These days, most books do not group the essences in this fashion anymore. Instead they are listed alphabetically, a cumbersome arrangement because one needs to plough through 38 essences in order to find something we need. Returning to Dr Bach's original groupings is a useful way to understand the essences and their relationship to each other in the system. It also offers a quick and effective way to identify and narrow our choices.

Since there are many books written on the indications of the flower essences, they will not be individually treated here. Instead, the focus in this chapter is to help readers appreciate and understand the significance and use of the seven groups. The 38 essences are presented in their individual categories, with the differences within a group highlighted to aid readers in their selection (Tables 1-7). All the essences in a particular category treat the same condition, but each addresses a specific cause, form or expression of that condition.

⊛ Broad And Versatile Application

In general the essences offer a number of benefits. They help to relieve stress because every single negative emotion and mental state has its negative effect on the physical system; it is stress on the body. The essences enable us to process and release these disturbing internal states.

Secondly, they bring the mind back into balance and perspective, so that life itself comes back into perspective. One recovers a mental and emotional clarity and calm to deal creatively and constructively with our individual challenges.

Thirdly, some use the system as a tool for personal transformation. Using the essences in this way can lead us on a journey of self-discovery. The essences dissolve obscurations; they open windows in the mind for us to see things about ourselves that we may have never seen before. They are therefore extremely helpful for those on a spiritual path, who may need assistance to work through negative traits and to develop certain virtues.

And then, of course, there are those who are physically ill. For them, the essences can take care of the psychogenic aspects of the illness. They relieve the fear, sadness, despondency or hopelessness that commonly accompany an illness. Fear, for example, is common in cancer patients. Even after successful surgery, therapy or when the cancer has gone into remission, the fear of recurrence lives on in many patients. This fear blocks the body's natural capacity to heal itself. By allowing negative emotions such as this to leave, the body can mobilize its resources effectively to engage fully in battling the disease. Proper healing can take place and the person can have a real chance of regaining full health.

Unlike other modalities, there are no circumscribed conditions for the use of the essences. Wherever there are human beings, there will be the challenges, issues and problems of human existence. In all cases, the essences can treat our 'diseased' reactions so that we can maintain an inner poise so crucial to healthy living. The message of Dr Bach goes beyond fixing problems as they arise; his philosophy points out to us that "a personality without conflict is immune to disease". By restoring internal harmony, we not only build immunity to physical illness but also reinstate emotional and mental balance, clarity and peace that are reflected externally in healthy, balanced relationships with others and the world at large. The key to healing the issues of life is to heal the individual at the center of that life, and the healing of one individual has far-reaching implications for the healing of the greater community.

[1] The Bach Flower Remedies: Illustrations and Preparations by Nora Weeks and Victor Bullen. Published by The C.W. Daniel Company Ltd, 1964, revised 1990.
[2] Cuba - Where Alternative Medicine Is Mainstream by Sara Altshul, Prevention Aug 2003 Vol. 55/No. 8.
[3] Quoted from Bach Flower Remedies to the Rescue by Gregory Vlamis. Published by Healing Arts Press, 1986, revised 1988, 1990.
[4] Flowers Soothe Savage Beasts by Denise Flaim, Newsday.com, June 27, 2000 page B15.
[5] Nature's Prozac by Harold Morrison, Nature's Health, May/June 1995.

Figure 1: The Seven Groups of Essences

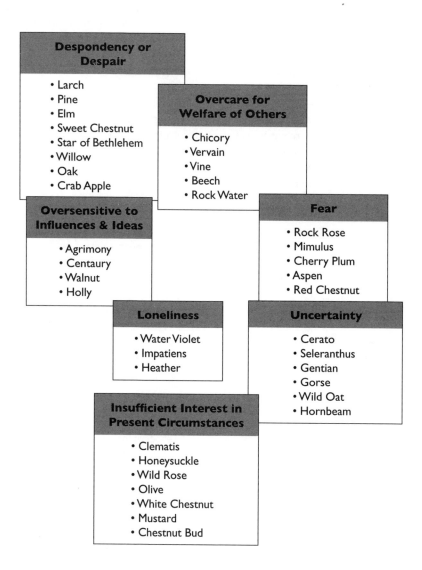

Despondency or Despair

- Larch
- Pine
- Elm
- Sweet Chestnut
- Star of Bethlehem
- Willow
- Oak
- Crab Apple

Overcare for Welfare of Others

- Chicory
- Vervain
- Vine
- Beech
- Rock Water

Oversensitive to Influences & Ideas

- Agrimony
- Centaury
- Walnut
- Holly

Fear

- Rock Rose
- Mimulus
- Cherry Plum
- Aspen
- Red Chestnut

Loneliness

- Water Violet
- Impatiens
- Heather

Uncertainty

- Cerato
- Seleranthus
- Gentian
- Gorse
- Wild Oat
- Hornbeam

Insufficient Interest in Present Circumstances

- Clematis
- Honeysuckle
- Wild Rose
- Olive
- White Chestnut
- Mustard
- Chestnut Bud

Group 1: Fear

There are **five** fear essences, each describing a distinctive cause and expression of fear.

Essence	Cause	Expression
Rock Rose	emergency and life-threatening situations such as accidents, natural disasters, nightmares or sudden fright	panic and terror, often accompanied by physical symptoms such as shaking, cold sweats, screaming; the nature of this fear is acute, escalated and extreme
Mimulus	issues of survival and existence	fear of worldly things related to everyday life – fear of life, death, pain, sickness, poverty, animals, height; in all cases, the objects of this fear are known to the sufferer
Cherry Plum	a mind under strain losing perspective, reason and control	fear of losing control of oneself and actual loss of control; this fear is irrational, impulsive and out of control and applies to the mental, emotional and physical
Aspen	vague, undefined, groundless fears and fears of the inexplicable and unknown	fear manifesting as an underlying uneasiness or anxiety, a sense of foreboding, an unpleasant expectancy of something bad, evil or disastrous to come
Red Chestnut	concern for loved ones that is blown out of proportion	overly fearful for loved ones; become anxious, worried and anticipate mishaps to befall those they care about

Group 2: Uncertainty

Uncertainty can express itself variedly as hesitance, doubt, indecision, vacillation, confusion and/or a lack of confidence in one's decision-making and decisions. The following **six** essences are indications for a variety of causes and expressions of uncertainty.

Essence	Cause	Expression
Cerato	uncertain because the person does not trust own judgement and decisions	needs and actively seeks affirmation, confirmation and assurance from others for the decisions they make; allows others' influence and advice to override one's own wisdom
Scleranthus	uncertain because the person cannot decide between two things	vacillates between one thing and the other; often feels stuck and caught in a dilemna
Gentian	uncertain of the outcome of an event or their effort	unduly discouraged and disheartened by setbacks and disappointments, and gives up easily
Gorse	uncertain there is use to try anymore	hopeless and despairing; sees the situation as useless and has given up the fight
Hornbeam	uncertain of their physical, mental or spiritual strength	mental weariness and boredom that delays action; procrastinates in routine areas of life
Wild Oat	uncertain of direction in life, immediate or long-term	dabbles and tries out many things in life but fails to find satisfaction and fulfillment; feels lost and confused

Group 3: Insufficient Interest in Present Circumstances

*This next category of **seven** essences describes mental or emotional states that take one's attention away from the present.*

Essence	Cause	Expression
Clematis	not present because they are wrapped in a mental world of imagination	outwardly drowsy and unaware, but mentally active and engaged in envisioning, wishing and hoping for better times in the future; sleeping, daydreams, fantasies are common
Honeysuckle	not present because they are trapped by past memories	positive memories bring nostalgia and longing for the past; unpleasant memories bring regrets and unrest over the past
Wild Rose	not present because they have no zest and interest in life	resigned and apathetic to their own life; take no initiative or make effort to improve their circumstances and well-being
Olive	not present because they are too exhausted physically, mentally and/or emotionally	the person runs out of fuel, has no or little energy to take care of daily life which becomes hard work for them
White Chestnut	not present because they are distracted by mental chatter	circling, repetitive unwanted thoughts that disturb mental peace and concentration
Mustard	not present because they are preoccupied with the melancholy that overcomes them	dark gloom and depression that descends and lifts without apparent reason; robs all interest and joy from the person
Chestnut Bud	not present because they are not observant and do not pay attention	make same mistakes over and over again because they fail to learn from the lessons of daily life

Group 4: Loneliness

These **three** types of characters often find themselves alone, either by choice and often not over time. Due to a pattern of continuous isolation from others, they suffer from loneliness compounded by an inability to relate to people. Their effects are evident in interactions with family members, intimate relationships, socially or at work. Here, loneliness is the end expression of these patterns.

Essence	Cause	Expression
Water Violet	suffers from a sense of separateness from others; underlying this is the feeling of being different, often in a superior way	alone and lonely because of a preference for one's own company; selective and picky about whom they interact with; dislikes and feels alone in crowds
Impatiens	suffers from an impatient nature that wants things done quickly and efficiently	alone and lonely at any task or work due to an inability to tolerate others' pace, methods and mistakes
Heather	suffers from a fear of being alone	loneliness drives them to self-absorption and at times obsession; they cling to anyone in company and talk incessantly about the thing they know best – themselves

Group 5: Oversensitive to Influences and Ideas

These **four** essences describe types who are easily affected, distracted and influenced by others and the environment.

Essence	Cause	Expression
Agrimony	overly sensitive to discord and conflict, wants peace at all cost	seeks distraction from external conflicts by accomodating and pacifying others, joking and adopting a jovial façade; seeks distraction from inner conflicts by becoming numb to one's own emotions and in some cases, using external substances or activities to accomplish this
Centaury	overly sensitive to what pleases others	easily affected by others' needs and wishes, likes and dislikes and quick to attend to them, in the process losing sight of their own life and purpose
Walnut	born with an innate and highly developed sensitivity	easily distracted from their own course in life by the influences of people, the times and the environment
Holly	suffers from a distorted oversensitivity	easily provoked by things that do not normally bother others; leads to quick irritation, hatred and malicious intent

Group 6: Despondency or Despair

The following group of **eight** describes different causes leading to despondency and/or despair.

Essence	Cause	Expression
Larch	feels inadequate in themselves	become despondent because of tendency to compare and feel inferior to others; lack confidence in own abilities, expect failure and stop themselves from trying and accomplishing
Pine	overly responsible for everyone and everything	become despondent from blaming and faulting themselves, even for others' mistakes; suffer from discontent, guilt and self-reproach
Elm	temporarily overwhelmed by the responsibilities they have taken on	become despondent from temporary feelings of inadequacy and loss of confidence in their ability and capacity to tackle the tasks at hand
Sweet Chestnut	mind and body taken to its utmost limits of endurance	expressive, unbearable anguish and despair that feels like total annihilation
Star of Bethlehem	bad news, traumatic events, losses or serious conditions	become despondent from shock, distress or grief
Willow	cannot accept adversity and misfortune in life	blame others and feel a victim of circumstances; become despondent from resentment and bitterness
Oak	a brave and stoic nature that does not give up	do not heed their own needs; become despondent when their body fails them and they become indisposed to fulfill their duties
Crab Apple	feeling unclean in body, feelings or thoughts	become despondent from perceived flaws in themselves

Group 7: Over-care for Welfare of Others

All the **five** characters in this group have one similarity: they are strong personalities who have a compelling desire to take care of others. However, the way they care becomes problematic when the tendency is to either dominate, interfere or influence in an unhealthy way.

Essence	Cause	Expression
Chicory	smothering, possessive and conditional love for others	overcare by overdoing and interfering in the lives of those they love, believing only they know the best for them
Vervain	strong will, zeal and convictions in their principles, views and ideas	overcare by trying to persuade and convert others to their way of thinking
Vine	possess great clarity, certainty and assurance in themselves	overcare by dominating others, dictating and directing them in their doings and lives
Beech	judgmental and intolerant	overcare by focusing in a negative way on the habits, idiosyncrasies or differences in others
Rock Water	strict, self-denying type who are hard masters on themselves	overcare by demanding themselves to be living examples of the ideals they embrace

Part II

*Understanding
Therapy and Usage*

This system of healing ... shows that it is our fears,

our cares, our anxieties ... that open the path

to the invasion of illness ... As the herbs heal

our fears, our anxieties, our worries,

our faults and failings ... then the disease,

no matter what it is, will leave us.

**Dr Edward Bach
Twelve Healers**

3

The Meaning of Therapy

The main obstacle people face when using the essences is a lack of understanding about this form of therapy. We must remember that for centuries now, medical science has consistently and insistently inculcated in us a mechanistic view of the body. Just as we send in a faulty automobile to the mechanic for repair or replacement, many of us would park our body in front of a doctor for him or her to fix. Much of the time, effort and money in medical research to this day are still focused on finding solutions for malfunctioning parts of the body.

Although this view has been eroded to some degree with the advent of complementary modalities of healing, it would take many more decades to undo what has already been deeply entrenched in the psyche of the masses. To understand how this view has permeated so much into our consciousness, we need only observe those who promote mind-body healing in the medical community yet do not necessarily use it themselves. Even those who offer mind-body healing are quick to feel fear when physical symptoms manifest, and eagerly adopt the same old familiar mechanistic solutions. In either case, there is no fundamental change in the view of the person.

The purpose of this chapter is to explore various misconceptions and clear away any confusion which may stop you from considering Bach Flower Essences as an option for your own healing. The more educated you are, the more conscious understanding and intention you can bring into the healing process, and the more rapidly you can get well.

🌸 Treat The Person, Not The Disease

The system of Bach Flower Essences is based solely on treating the person; that is, treating the individual's passing moods, mental outlook and personality type. **Passing moods** are temporary states of mind. Perhaps we wake up one morning feeling unexpectedly gloomy. A couple of drops of the *Mustard* essence would help to dispel the melancholy for the day. After a spat of intense hard work, we may find ourselves exhausted and easily overwhelmed by a simple task. Taking *Olive* can revive our vitality and *Elm* can help restore confidence in our capacity. The sudden shock of receiving bad news is another passing state and this one can be taken care by *Star of Bethlehem*.

Mental outlook is our attitude and habitual perception. It refers to the way a person views life, others and the self. This can range from perceiving oneself as separate and isolated (a *Water Violet* trait), to having a victim mentality (*Willow* tendency), to believing that one is powerless to change things (*Wild Rose*). **Personality traits** are long-term habitual tendencies and patterns of behavior that we often use to describe a person. For example, we can describe someone as strongly principled (*Vervain* type), another as critical and intolerant, picking faults with a sharp tongue (*Beech*) and a bully who forces his or her way with things (*Vine*).

Therefore, in trying to help yourself and others, the questions to ask are: What emotions are disturbing my mind at the moment? Am I depressed, sad, feeling hopeless or lonely? What complaints do I usually have with life, with people or even myself? Do I resent life as unfair, feel inadequate and less than others in many ways? Do I relate to myself with disdain and despair? What are the patterns of thoughts and behavior I have come to identify as who I am or that others commonly use to describe me? Am I a stoic, a loner, or an incessant talker? Do others call me timid and shy or strong and domineering? Or am I seen as rigid and inflexible or weak and confused?

Whether you are a Bach practitioner or a lay person, it is this type of information that provides the indicators for identifying the correct essences. The physical complaints become irrelevant because *different mental and*

emotional causes can bring about the same physical symptoms. We can see this from the example of three children who have come down with a flu. Little Tom is grumpy and whiny, Beth is sleepy and drowsy, and Martha is throwing her temper tantrums. Although all three children suffer from similar symptoms, each is treated for their individual temperament. Accordingly, *Chicory* is given to Tom, *Clematis* to Beth and *Cherry Plum* to Martha. A second illustration of the same concept is given in Figure (2).

A Case of Insomnia

When a patient visits a doctor and complains of insomnia, the doctor would ordinarily prescribe a sleeping pill. In the Bach system, there is no single essence for insomnia. Therapy begins with the practitioner and client exploring the emotional-mental states that are preventing the individual from getting a good night's sleep. In the examples given below, appropriate essences are used to address different mental/emotional causes even though all individuals concerned are experiencing the same physical problem of sleeplessness.

- I cannot sleep because I am worried sick about my children.   Red Chestnut
- I cannot sleep because I am so nervous and worried about my financial situation now that I am jobless.   *Mimulus*
- I cannot sleep because the day's conversations and events keep going round and round in my head.   White Chestnut
- I cannot sleep because I feel so bad and guilty for letting my whole team down.   Pine
- I cannot sleep because I am overcome with grief at the loss of my parents.   Star of Bethlehem
- I cannot sleep because I am mad and resent my boss for picking on me in the office.   Willow
- I cannot sleep because I miss home and wish my family and friends were here with me.   Honeysuckle
- I cannot sleep because I cannot decide whether to leave this relationship or not.   Scleranthus
- I cannot sleep because I am not used to these new and unfamiliar surroundings.   Walnut

Figure (2)

One of the most difficult things to accomplish in this therapy is to help those in need to make that internal shift from a fixation on physical symptoms to a focus on mental-emotional events as a pathway to health. Dr Bach's message appears simple on the surface but, without exploring its deeper and broader implications, is difficult to grasp and fully integrate. Invariably after a talk, one or two members of the audience would approach and ask, "So, what would you use to get rid of calcium deposits? Which essences would you recommend for stomach ulcer? What can I give to my friend who has just been diagnosed with cancer?"

It is easy to understand why this message is so difficult to take root. We have been immersed in decades, even centuries of a medical culture that keeps pointing us to the symptoms as the source for answers. In fact, the current practice and understanding of diseases is to classify them according to physical symptoms. This classification defines diagnosis and treatment. We are trained to focus primarily on body parts, names of illnesses, failing biological mechanisms, and to correlate and counteract physical problems with specific chemical compounds or medical technology. Not understanding the deep and profound connection between the physical and essential aspects of ourselves, we treat the experience of the body as separate from who we are. Since this is the pervasive mindset of the world, most of us instinctively gravitate towards it even when we are exposed to alternative ways of thinking.

Such views and practice of medicine have taken our attention away from the true indicators of disease. So much so that when some clients are asked to relate their mental or emotional states, they can be stumped and do not know how to proceed. We are not taught to pay attention to how we are feeling and thinking; least of all to connect them to our illness. Certain cultures, in particular the Asian, promote the Agrimony trait. Entertaining and expressing emotions can be taboo in a family, a sign of selfishness, weakness or ingratitude and often forcibly discouraged or critically brushed aside. True individual expression is frowned upon even to these days. This is a cultural pattern that has come down through generations; it does not go away simply by mimicking western ways. Children who have learned to suppress, deny and ignore how they feel are most likely to grow up into adults who do the same. Some may reach a point where they have little access to their emotions and experiences, and honestly cannot provide the information so necessary for therapy to proceed.

As a practitioner, I have the good fortune of working with clients from two very different cultures. Asians in general have greater difficulty in connecting with themselves than their Western counterparts. Many continue to talk about the pain, the body, the medication and treatment even though they have come to a therapy that deals specifically with mental and emotional states. I have witnessed my clients' struggle with their inner experiences either out of fear, uncertainty or confusion, and this applies even to the most educated. Those who have lost touch with how they feel can be unsure and confused when asked to describe their emotional experiences. The fear of betrayal arises when the issue is dissatisfaction or unhappiness with someone close to them. Information is withheld and this prohibits an accurate assessment. This problem stems from a common confusion about 'engaging' and 'acknowledging' a negative emotion or attitude; they are not the same thing. When we engage in the anger that rises in us, we act it out through some malicious thoughts, harsh words or physical action to harm or hurt. But to recognize the destructive nature of the anger and to acknowledge the problem is healthy. Without this first step, a person cannot even begin to do the necessary work to become free from it.

This obstacle is also a particularly common one amongst those who follow a spiritual tradition. They fear the darker emotions in themselves and often seek to suppress them because it is not spiritually right or correct to feel that way. They try to avoid, ignore and deny but these energetic patterns do not simply disappear under a new cloak of 'good habits' layered over them. They will remain as long as they are unattended. The healthy practitioner understands the difference between acknowledging and engaging in a negative emotion or attitude. By looking honestly at these emotions – the anger, jealousy, pride, attachment and often less than lofty motivation for their spiritual activities – they can learn a great deal about themselves and know where to put their effort in eliminating the less desirable and cultivating the desirable. The path becomes authentic and freeing.

Knowing these hurdles in advance does not automatically remove them, but becoming aware is the first step to begin work. Therapy can begin as long as the client is willing to acknowledge and confront even the obstacles to therapy.

Disease Our Teacher

We have been taught to fear physical disease, to see it as an enemy, to fight it, beat it back, or run away from it. Of course, it will initially seem frightening to abandon our focus on physical symptoms when they are the most apparent signs of illness. However, they are essentially only signals of deeper unrest, and the emotions of fear, anger and resentment surrounding illness are themselves great impediments to healing.

Dr Bach offers us an alternative way to relate to physical disease that is both healthy and freeing. He said in his book *Heal Thyself,* "Disease, though apparently so cruel, is in itself beneficent and for our good and, if rightly interpreted, will guide us to our essential faults. Suffering is a corrective to point out a lesson which by other means we have failed to grasp, and never can it be eradicated until that lesson is learnt."

All sickness is a sign of spiritual dis-ease, an indication that a person is not living in alignment with their deepest spiritual reality. Disease is like a teacher awakening us to the knowledge of where we have gone astray and the possibility of becoming free of our errors. It serves to alert us to the danger of being mistaken in the way we are. Therefore we should not fear but instead welcome the lessons to be learned and make the necessary correction in order to be well again. When this true cause of illness is removed, it is possible to eradicate the physical ailment. This is a message of hope for all of us.

Physician Heal Thyself

By conventional definition, the healer has always been seen as the doctor, the herbalist, the chiropractor and so on. Because of this concept, people believe that only these individuals have the power to make them well. In the process, they dis-empower and, in some cases, conveniently absolve themselves of any responsibility in their own healing. If they do not get well, it is the practitioner who is not good or the technique that is not good, or the medicine that is not good. What follows is an endless hunt for the best healer with the best technique and the best medicine. Such activities only distract from the real cause of disease and healing which is within.

The power to heal is largely in the hands of the individual. As soon as we become aware of this, we have the choice to use this power. Clients often come to me wanting me to fix them. They do this because they do not understand the underlying philosophy of this therapy. With modalities that treat the person rather than the disease, success is unlikely without the client's desire to learn, to change and to act. The unconditional desire to heal is already half the battle won. I say 'unconditional' because many clients have conditions for their healing. They want the pain, the illness to go away but are not willing to look at where it is coming from. They want to be healed but have no time to attend to the healing process. They want their problems to go away but do not want to look at how their attitudes are contributing to them. Relapses and slow progress are common because the fundamental understanding has never been established and the fundamental cause has never been eliminated.

Holding Pure View

Effective therapy also requires another paradigm shift within the client as well as the practitioner. This one is to focus on innate spiritual perfection as the reality of the individual, that every person who comes in need of help is fundamentally whole. What they need is assistance to eliminate the negative emotions and traits that obstruct their natural and unique expression. The role of the practitioner and, for that matter, anyone using the essences to help another is to reinstate mental and emotional homeostasis or balance. We are not fixing what is bad, what has gone wrong. We are focused on unveiling and freeing true expression, on helping the person to reconnect with their essential nature.

I do not have children who come and seek help on their own accord. It is always the parents who either perceive them to have a problem or to be the problem. The common practice of attaching faults to the child compounds and confuses the issue. One mother in Singapore called to tell me she could not recognize her son anymore. She was in shock and wondered what I had done to him. This was a 9-year-old boy who was out of control, terrorizing his younger sisters and mother, and then went through a rather dramatic transformation in a matter of a week on the essences. I had to assure the mother that this was her 'real son'.

Two other mothers from Berkeley had a similar issue. One of them commented that she and her partner were wondering if they were 'doping' their 3-year-old girl with flower essences. They were glad that she had turned into a sweet thing but the transformation was just too unbelievable! Another parent was reluctant to continue therapy because she did not want to 'fix' her son and alter his personality. I had to explain to her that whether she is fixing or not fixing the child has to do with her intention, not the form of therapy. The essences do not change the child's basic nature; instead they help to clear away the obstacles for this essence to come forth and for him to be happy and therefore healthy. The negative emotions and traits we see in children are not who they are. These are the actual illnesses that we as adults can help the child to overcome, knowing and holding at all times their natural beauty and perfection. By viewing things this way, we would have more compassion for the undesirable traits we see in our children and in ourselves, traits that we would normally criticize and reject. Then, by using the appropriate essences with proper understanding, we can gradually eliminate them.

Adults can also make the same mistake with themselves. Once I offered a friend a solution to his problems with the flower essences. His immediate concern was: "Am I going to change after taking them?" He wanted his indecision to go away but he did not want to change his personality in order to accomplish this. This is how unconscious we normally are. It did not occur to him that it would be contradictory to want his indecisiveness to go away without a change in his 'indecisive' personality. There are many clients who, like this friend, face the same predicament – they want to get well but they do not want to change.

This resistance comes as before from falsely identifying themselves with their fears, uncertainties, insecurities and confusion. Their personalities do change with therapy; but their true nature does not. Change also raises the fear of the unknown in some. It is often sufficient to help the client become aware of the contradictions in their intention to help them move past the fear. But even if this is not enough, working with the appropriate essences will eliminate the objections and pave the way to a smoother healing process.

The Role Of Conscious Intent

Dr Bach spoke of "developing the opposing virtues" as part of therapy. What did he mean by this? In essence, it is to make conscious effort to cultivate the opposite of what we are suffering from. For example, if you are a fearful person and each time you react to a person or event with fear, you habituate yourself to the fear. Over time, the energy grows in strength and the person becomes increasingly fearful and, at the worst, reaches a state where they can become paralyzed by panic attacks. If the person is developing the opposing virtue, then each time the fear presents itself, he or she consciously disengages from it and instead musters the courage to act. In this way, the old habit is slowly broken and a new habit formed. This element of conscious effort speeds up the process of healing considerably.

As part of the therapy offered, I often counsel my clients on ways to develop this opposing virtue. For instance, if the client has a Pine tendency of blaming and reproaching themselves, one way to cut the pattern of negative self-talk would to draw up a contract with themselves to stop this constant self-disparagement. In addition to taking the essences, they practice this mindful restraint daily. By choosing to disengage from the habit, they stop it from increasing in strength. By taking the essences, they allow the vibrations of this pattern to be flushed out of their system. This two-pronged approach constitutes a complete therapy.

Developing some kind of detachment and space between your conscious will and unconscious patterns of thoughts, speech and action is therefore useful. Clients who have done meditation or are used to inner spiritual work have the advantage of adding this element to their therapy and usually see rapid and profound progress. For those who do not engage in such practices, spending some quiet time each day for and by yourself is a good start.

Obstacles In Therapy

How you approach your own healing is determined by the very traits that bring you into therapy. The *Impatiens* type will want quick results; they have no patience to understand the essences or their healing process. They leave therapy when they do not get immediate results. The *Gentian* personality is dismayed by the slightest setback and may give up early on in therapy. The *Vervain*, with an appetite for over-effort, may adopt 'the more the better' attitude and put themselves under the care of a platoon of healing practitioners. The *Cerato* is unsure of progress; they need others to confirm, assure and influence them in their choice of therapies. Uncertainty plagues them in all aspects of life right down to their inner experience. When asked if they experience any change with the essences, they are unlikely to provide any definite feedback.

Vine clients want to run the consultation session and dictate the outcome of therapy. This demanding attitude can obstruct the practitioner from effectively helping them. They are unable to surrender to therapy or allow their healing process to unfold. Their frustration and desire to leave comes because of their fixation on preconceived outcomes. *Chicory* clients may unconsciously not want to get well. Illness can be a useful ally to them, bringing the attention and support they seek from loved ones or the practitioner to whom they have formed an attachment. *Willow* types begrudge the benefits of therapy, make ungrateful patients and clients and seldom want to be responsible for their own healing or the way their lives have turned out. Another type that tends to overstay in therapy is the lonely *Heather* who needs someone to listen to them.

If you are helping someone, it is important to eliminate these obstacles as soon as they come up with the appropriate essences. Otherwise these very same traits will distract the person and deter them from experiencing the full efficacy of the flower essences.

❁ Handling The Skeptic

The skeptic's contention is: "Prove to me before I will believe." Their disbelief forbids them to experience anything they cannot yet comprehend, and can deny them the opportunity to use the essences and become well. Most skeptics are also proud of their skepticism, and therefore see no reason in letting go of an attitude that does not always serve them well.

A woman in an audience once remarked, "How could you as a trained pharmacist believe in such things?" Well, beliefs come and go; we change them the same way we change fashion in cars or clothes or hairstyles. This applies even to medical information that has been proven, only to be disproved later. The most recent example is the benefits of HRT (hormone replacement therapy) for menopausal women. That was a fashionable medical belief at one time, and now recent studies have shown that prolonged use poses significant health risks.

There is therefore nothing holy about beliefs that we have to stay loyal to them; neither is there any virtue in clinging on to the belief of non-belief. Oftentimes we are victims of our own skepticism. We unconsciously choose to believe in things that keep us in our comfort zones; we dislike being challenged or our minds to be rocked too violently by new discoveries and views. Of course, it is wise and intelligent to carefully examine new bodies of knowledge presented to us. But at some point, to truly know their efficacy, one has to apply and use this knowledge and assess through one's own experience. In the case of the essences, this means taking them for the ills we are suffering. For those who have done so and experienced the benefits, no one can ever deny or take away their experiences. This must be the strongest proof for anyone seeking proof.

⊛ Finding The Appropriate Helper

A normal visit to a doctor does not present itself as a problem for most of us. We can talk about our body parts rather detachedly; but when it comes to describing our emotions and mental states, we identify more closely with them and it is not uncommon for people to become intensely personal about their issues. This form of therapy therefore requires a great deal more trust between helper and helpee. Without a safe and trusting environment, it is difficult for a person to open up and speak about their inner experiences.

If you wish to work with a practitioner, it is therefore essential to find one you can trust and have confidence in. Otherwise the lack of connection and resonance in your relationship can become an obstacle to therapy too. If you are helping someone else, it is important to humbly acknowledge when appropriate that we may not be the right person to help that individual and withdraw graciously. Otherwise, we can exacerbate or become part of the problem. The person can resist therapy because of *our* attitudes, behavior and intentions towards them. This is especially a case to be put forward for family members. Family members have a longer history with each other. Over time they have become habituated to certain perceptions and conceptions of each other. Therefore they are less likely to be detached and unbiased in their assessment, making their help more uncomfortable and sometimes unpleasant to receive. In such instances, a third party may be the more effective choice to deliver the help needed.

Practitioners and helpers bring their own personality traits and habitual attitudes and emotions into the assistance they offer. A *Beech* family member or therapist who has not resolved their own critical and judgmental mode of perception, speech and body language can do a great deal of damage to the person they are trying to help. So much negativity is loaded onto the individual who is already suffering that it will most likely make matters worse. A *Vine* parent or counselor, who does not have an active program to keep themselves in check and balance, could be overriding their children or clients in life decisions and choices. They disempower the other in their healing process. The *Chicory* type disempowers by encouraging neediness and weakness in others. They enjoy being needed and being the stronger one who knows what is best. Such co-dependency bodes ill for a healthy relationship and proper healing.

These examples are brought up to raise the awareness that many elements contribute to a successful healing, beginning with the attitudes we bring into therapy, our working relationship with the practitioner or person helping us, and our own desire to confront the true cause of the problems and to take action. This is the case for all forms of therapies, not just the Bach Flower Essences. This simple mindfulness of the multi-faceted nature of healing allows us to foresee potential obstacles and to sidestep unnecessary hindrances on our journey back to health, thereby offering a better chance of accessing the full potential of the therapy in question.

4

Working with the Essences

This chapter is designed to guide you through the process of choosing, preparing and using the essences. Although the system offers us an extremely easy way to treat ourselves, the information and tips collected here from various sources and practical experience will help you to know what to do and what to expect.

Choosing Your Essences

When choosing essences, it is recommended that you try to identify the root cause of your problem and then the appropriate essence. The less essences we put into a formula, the better it is because we can then bear clearly in mind the mental-emotional habits we are working on and the changes to expect. The recognition of change is important to assess our progress and to encourage us in our healing process. However, since we are all multi-faceted individuals, it is frequently the case that more than one essence may be required for any given situation in which case, as many as six to seven may be combined for use.

To clarify your selection, you can make use of books or available consumer literature and aids such as reference guides, recommendation chart, wall chart, pamphlets, flower cards and selection wheels. Some are free of charge, including a questionnaire compiled by Nelsonbach. Going through the questionnaire is an easy way to put a preliminary selection in place. For clients who have difficulty articulating their problems, I sometimes use this exercise to help them get started. However, this is not a foolproof method. Some people are too shy or embarrassed to indicate what are perceived as 'bad' aspects of themselves, and therefore inadvertently omit them. Besides, we each have our blind spots which can make it difficult to see certain things about ourselves. When this happens, it is useful to seek feedback from someone who knows you well. We must also be aware that the three questions listed per essence do not fully describe the indication and scope of that particular essence. Individuals also relate to different descriptions of the same essence. So although the questionnaire is helpful, it should not be relied upon completely.

> *The website www.bachfloweressences.co.uk offers a variety of helpful information: descriptions of the 38 essences, an online tutorial, remedy chooser which is an interactive questionnaire, a place to download your favorite Bach leaflets, and information on training programs.*

For more information, you can refer to a basic book such as *The 38 Bach Flower Essences*. This contains a more detailed description of each of the 38 essences and Rescue Remedy, the emotional and mental conditions for which each is needed together with the positive potential of the flowers. It also provides instruction on how to use the essences. Dr Bach's succinct description of the essences in *The Twelve Remedies and Others* is another important reference. Other useful books are listed in the Appendix, and they may be found in your local library or bookstores.

When we first familiarize ourselves with the essences, it may seem that a great many applies to us. This is a common initial reaction from the audience. Once, after a public talk at a library, a woman came up to me and insisted she needed all 38 essences and I had not even covered all 38! People readily and instinctively identify with the emotional and mental traits that are described because they are so universal. They respond because the essences speak of familiar daily human experiences.

There are a number of reasons why you would not need all 38. At any one moment, it is rare for a person to simultaneously experience all 38 states described by the entire system. It is definitely possible that you may use all 38 over a period of time, but not all at the same time. Secondly, putting too many essences together clouds the issues. Part of the healing is for you to develop self-awareness and understanding. When we are taking a few essences and know exactly what we are trying to overcome, we become more aware of those aspects of ourselves and learn to consciously move towards the opposite virtue. When we use 38, we no longer have a clear idea of what is working or not working for us and therefore cannot grow in this self-knowledge. Thirdly, Dr Bach himself had tried using all 38 in combination, had not found it useful and did not recommend it.

It is easy to be confused about the essences we need because we are not in the habit of assessing our emotions nor are we trained to work with them. People respond to their emotions in many different ways. Some are afraid of them and spend a lifetime blocking them out. Others are too embarrassed and ashamed and try to hide them. Then there are those who react with criticism and reproach and others who dwell too much on negativity and turn forlorn and depressed. As mentioned before, it is of utmost importance that we stop identifying and engaging with our habitual patterns of negative thoughts or emotions. We are not our anger, confusion, depression or fear, just as the clouds are not the sky. A degree of personal detachment is crucial for an accurate assessment of what we need.

There are, however, instances in life when too many issues confront us. Here are some guidelines for those who need help to narrow down their choices:

(1) **Treat the acute and immediate**. A person under severe stress can manifest certain symptoms such as feeling overwhelmed, showing exhaustion, or at the brink of a nervous breakdown. Take care of these first with *Elm* (overwhelmed), *Olive* (exhaustion), *Cherry Plum* (nervous strain) and *Rescue Remedy* (stress). After the first phase of treatment, you

can move on to investigate the causes that led to such a situation.

(2) **Prioritize your needs**. Ask yourself what are the most important things you have to address at this point in time, and use the relevant essences to do so. Leave the less important issues for a later time.

(3) **Base your choice on your type**. Ask yourself: "How would I describe myself as a person? What is my usual response to stress? Do I lose control, do I become fearful, or do I become very unsure of myself?" Questions like this will lead you to a few core imbalances that can be treated easily with the right essences. Taking care of these core traits will keep in check their peripheral expressions.

How To Prepare

The essences are currently available in 10 and 20 ml bottles of stock concentrates. You do not need to take them neat from the stock solutions unless nothing else is available. All you need is a minute quantity and the way to obtain this depends on whether you are addressing passing moods or longer-term traits.

Comments on Intuitive Methods

Some individuals do not choose essences by relying on a knowledge of them; instead they use other means such as intuitively reaching out for the bottles, dowsing with a pendulum or using flower cards. This is not encouraged as the primary method of selection, although it does not mean that you cannot use them to confirm your selection. The main concern about such methods is that they bypass an important learning process for the individual. Final healing is experienced only when the person understands how they have gone astray in relationship to themselves and others. They understand the cause on a conscious level and with intent, make the decision to abandon such traits. Developing this healthy discriminating wisdom is essential for healing to be complete. For this reason, Dr Bach himself had said that all we need is healthy human judgment to use the essences well.

For emergencies or passing states, put two drops (four drops for Rescue Remedy) into a glass of water and sip at regular intervals until relief is obtained. If there is no water available, put neat into the mouth from the stock bottle. At times you may hear of someone who reported no effect after taking Rescue Remedy. Most likely, it is because the person had only taken one or two doses. In acute conditions, it is necessary to dose frequently, as often as every 5-15 min, in order to experience full relief.

For longer-term conditions, prepare a bottle with your own personal mix of essences. This bottle has been variedly referred to as a *treatment bottle, dosage bottle, mixing bottle,* or *personal formula* but they all mean the same thing.

Procedure for preparing a personal formula:

1. Fill a 30 ml bottle with glass dropper three-quarter full with bottled spring or mineral water.

2. Put two drops each of the chosen essences; four drops for Rescue Remedy if you are including this as well. Rescue Remedy counts as one essence.

3. Cap the bottle and tap gently against the palm to mix.

4. To dose, deliver four drops of the solution into the mouth.

If the climate is too hot, adding a preservative helps to keep the water stable for the duration of the bottle. A teaspoon of brandy, cider vinegar or glycerin is generally sufficient. Be sensitive in your choice of preservatives. For infants or individuals who are either alcohol-sensitive or opposed to taking it for religious reasons, do not use any alcoholic preservative. They should also be made aware that there will always be a tiny amount of alcohol in any formula because the stock concentrates are preserved in 27% alcohol. The residual taste of the alcohol in the formula can be masked by mixing the essences in juice or other beverages but if they still object to its presence, offer them alternative ways of using the essences (see Topical Application).

The bottle can also be kept cool in the refrigerator. This is convenient for the parent who is dosing the child, but otherwise it is more practical to keep the bottle with you for convenient dosing. Avoid touching the glass dropper tip to your tongue, teeth, lips or any other surface so that you do not contaminate the solution. If you do so, flush it under hot running water before returning to the bottle. Contamination is rare but easily detectable because the solution will taste unpleasant or growths can be seen floating in it. If this happens, discard the solution. The potency of the essences remains unchanged by the contamination but it is not a good idea to take in bad water. Continue dosing until you finish the formula.

One dosage bottle lasts between 1-3 weeks depending on how frequently the essences are taken. The minute dilution required makes the essences an economical form of therapy. Stock concentrates can last for years although, as you continue to use the essences and healing takes place, the essences needed will change over time.

⚛ Taking The Essences

• Why must the essences be dosed so often?

Unlike pharmaceutical and herbal preparations, the essences are not dose-dependent. They act to return our system to balance. Four drops of the dilution prepared is the effective dose to effect a change. Translated into practice, this means that taking eight drops does not double the effect of four drops. Instead, the return to balance depends on *how often* we take the effective dose. In this therapy, we do not speak of increasing dosage but of increasing dosing frequency.

The minimum recommended dosing is four times a day; once in the morning so the essences can help set the energy for the day; the other before sleep since disharmonies have been known to release in dreams. The other two doses are to be spread out evenly throughout the day. In fact, you need to dose as often as needed. What this means is to dose as frequently as you want or like, feel drawn or compelled to do so. The body takes to that which brings it into balance; therefore if the formula is right, you will find yourself reaching out for the essences. When that happens, it is perfectly fine to follow your impulses.

Most people, however, are new to this form of therapy and relate to the essences the way they would to medications, so are cautious of under-dosing, overdosing, side effects, interactions and the way they administer the doses. When asked to dose as frequently as needed, they do not know how. Clients find it easier to follow instructions than to intuitively come up with their own dosing program. For this reason, I have had to ask my clients to use as often as every two hours, every hour or every half-hour depending on the severity of the condition or the strength of that state. The more severe the condition and the stronger the emotional-mental pattern, the higher is the recommended frequency.

There is a belief that you need to take the essences one month for each year that you suffer from that condition. My own experiences with clients have shown that it is possible to circumvent this by increasing the dosing frequency. At four doses four times a day, a 64-yr-old client perceived no noticeable effects for months. It was only his tenacity and faith that kept him on therapy. Finally when he was asked to dose every half hour, he felt a change within a week. The changes were obvious: a brighter and softer face and eyes, and a renewed connection to himself.

This system is completely safe. There can be no danger of overdosing. When the system reaches balance, the essences no longer have an effect and you would not want to take them anymore. Similarly, those who have a tendency to miss doses need not be unduly worried. The only harm done is to delay your own healing. There is no need to make up for the missed dose by doubling the next. It does not work this way.

• **Can it be taken with food, or before or after food?**
The essences are energy extracts that act directly on the subtle energy

system of our body. Because they are not material in nature, there would be no interaction with substances such as food or medications. Hence it is not important whether they are taken with or without food. With infants, each dose can be put directly into baby food or the milk bottle; with pets, in their food or water.

• Are there drug interactions with the essences?
One of the dangers of pharmaceutical products is interaction with each other that can either potentiate or nullify their effects. Some drug interactions have caused death in patients. The beauty of the essences is that they cannot interfere or interact with any other treatment because the energy of the flowers acts on the energetic, not material aspect of the person. As a result, they are a proven helpful adjunct therapy to the healing modalities that do act on the substantial level. In some cases, use of the essences has enabled the patient to stop or decrease drug intake. A medical doctor in Seattle resorted to prescribing himself a sedative because he was having problems sleeping, which in turn interfered with his work. After one bottle of essences, he was able to sleep better and reduce his sedative dose by half.

• Will the essences cause psychological dependence?
Parents are readily alarmed when they see how well their children take to the essences. They fear that their children will develop a dependence on them. There is really no cause to fear. Once internal balance is achieved, you or your child will naturally wean yourselves off the essences and there will be no more desire to take them.

Another common concern amongst parents is that their child will swing to the other extreme. For instance, they may fear that their strong, domineering son may turn into a weakling after he has finished with Vine. This is not possible. The essences can only return the system to balance; they cannot over-balance.

• Must we finish the entire bottle?

It is advisable to finish the entire bottle before gauging your progress with the essences. If a formula works well, I often advise clients to take a second bottle of the same formula to consolidate the effects. It is, however, equally possible that an individual could be going through a phase of rapid change and that the formula they need changes by the week or even by the day. In this case, it is easier to prepare the formula on an as-needed basis, directly into a glass of water, than to prepare a different dosage bottle daily.

• How do we know if we need to continue taking?

It is easy. If you are suffering from depression and that depression has not lifted completely, you need to continue. In my practice, I find most adults too eager to take themselves and their children prematurely off therapy and then wonder why they have a 'relapse'. With some patience, you can completely eliminate an undesirable trait with the correct essence. What used to irritate, frighten or stress you stops having that effect on you; the intolerance, the procrastination, the feelings of inadequacy can completely cease given time. The essences are not band-aids, they are curative in nature. The effects are permanent but to achieve this takes desire and diligence. This point is especially important to remember when we are helping children because it can make a big difference to a long life ahead.

There are fans of technology who may demand a more objective measure of change from the use of essences. Just as we measure our blood pressure and count blood cells, we want machines to tell us if we are happy or sad, angry or depressed. This is a redundant endeavor because *feeling* and *thinking* and *perceiving* are human experiences. It would be very sad for mankind if there does come a day when we are so disconnected from ourselves that we no longer know what we are experiencing.

• How long do we have to use the essences?

In general, you can discontinue when you experience relief and the condition stabilizes. How long this actually takes depends very much on the individual because each one of us responds to the essences quite differently. Some are more sensitive than others, or they may have worked at a particular issue for a long time and, like a ripe fruit about to fall from the tree, that pattern is ready to leave. A Catholic sister took one dose of the essences and immediately felt a change in her body. One week on the formula and her constipation of many years never returned. Others with deep-seated distress and fears may need to take them longer to experience noticeable relief.

Passing moods would take a much shorter time to go away than personality traits. A younger person would need less therapy than an elderly person. Children respond very well to the essences because their mental-emotional patterns are fairly fresh and easy to release. The same patterns can be deeply ingrained through habituation in adults, and progressively so with age.

In actuality, each person defines his or her own meaning and goal for healing and therefore the length of therapy. To the executive who simply wants to get rid of his migraine so it does not interfere with his work, when the migraine is gone, his healing is complete. To the housewife seeking help for issues with her husband, when that relationship shifts for the better, her healing is complete. For those using this work to aid their spiritual practice or as a tool for personal growth – essentially a life-long endeavor – it is more likely to be regular and ongoing for a while. In general, I notice that my clients eventually reach a threshold of stability. When this happens, it is time to wean yourself off therapy. From then on, you can space your use of the essences further apart or use them on an as-needed basis. The other option is to develop new longer-term goals and carry on working.

❁ Topical Application

The skin is the largest organ in the body. Its large surface area allows rapid entry of external agents, including the essences. Because the energy body extends beyond the physical, this form of administering the essences is extremely effective since they are applied close to the site of imbalance.

Topical application to the pulse points at the wrists, behind the ears, on the lips is useful when the person is unconscious or objects to the slightest intake of alcohol. It is equally effective if not more so. Experiences with my clients reveal that the vibrations of negative attitudes and emotions can be generalized, localized or both. When it is localized, it creates disturbance in a specific area of the body. With clients who show physical distress, I commonly instruct them to take the essences orally and to apply doses directly to the body area manifesting those symptoms. Rescue Remedy is often used in this way. When one has a serious fall, you can apply the cream to the cuts and bruises and take the liquid to ease the shock at the same time. Using the essences in this combined way has proven to speed up the release of the negative energies, allowing rapid healing to take place. In his days, Dr Bach was fond of using compresses – towels soaked in solutions of essences – on the parts showing physical symptoms for, I suspect, the same reason.

There are other methods of topical application. One of my favorites is to spray a solution of essences into a room to clear the energy of the space, onto plants that need some reviving, or directly onto linen, clothes or the body. The essences can also be added to massage oil for a massage with a difference, or mixed with body lotion and face cream for personal care. They can also be put into a bath for a relaxing or revitalizing soak. The ways to administer the essences are limited only by our imagination.

The creative use of the essences becomes especially important for children. Parents can afford to be more playful so that dosing becomes fun and enjoyable for the child. Learn to work with your child: she may like to take the drops directly from the bottle, or he may like them applied to the head, or for others, you may have to slip it into their water bottle, juice, milk or beverage, or spray on the pillow or clothes. Do not let yourself be limited by any obstacle in administering the essences. Please allow your imagination to solve the problem for you.

✿ What To Expect

There are a number of things to look for when taking the essences. By knowing what to expect, we can better understand the process and eliminate unnecessary fear and interruption in our own healing.

1. No Response

When a person reports no effects after taking the essences, check up on the following:

✓ **Check compliance.** *Are they taking the essences and properly?*

Patient compliance is as big a problem with the essences as with conventional medication. I have known clients who take them less than the recommended four doses per day, or take them sporadically for a day or two here and there. Of course, it will take a longer time to notice change this way.

✓ **Check essences.** *Are they taking the right essences?*

Individuals who are uncommunicative, awkward or even guilty about expressing some harbored thoughts or feelings can provide insufficient or even misleading information. If you or the person you are helping is experiencing this difficulty, it is helpful to understand or explain the difference between *acknowledging* and *engaging* as discussed in the previous chapter. Acknowledgment is healthy; it paves the way for therapy to begin.

✓ **Check awareness.** *Is the client aware of changes?*

Oftentimes changes come but in the busyness of life, people do not notice them. One simple way to check this is to go over what the person said before and ask whether they have noticed any difference with each issue raised. This process usually helps them to recognize the changes more easily.

✓ **Check attitude.** *Does the individual type have hidden agendas?*

A person may want to exercise power (*Vine*), prove a point (*Vervain*), draw attention (*Chicory*), unconsciously keep their problems, afraid to get well because they have to face life again (*Mimulus*), or to take responsibility for themselves (*Willow*). These are some reasons why people do not want to get well. They are real issues we have to handle skillfully when people are resisting change. Skill here could mean finding a timely moment to bring it to their attention, or presenting the issue in a more palatable way. We can know how best to do this by putting ourselves in the shoes of the other.

2. Cleansing Effects

There are no side effects in the use of the essences; however there are cases where someone can experience discomfort when using them. When we take the essences, we are flushing our system with the positive vibrations of the flowers and in that process, release the vibrations of troubling emotions or attitudes. As they move out of the body, these negative vibrations express themselves. If it is anger, we will feel anger. If it is grief, we will feel the sadness.

These seeming side effects can manifest as physical or emotional distress. Physical examples would be cold, rash, upset stomach, headache, and diarrhea or even in one case, bad breath. The expressions are varied. Sometimes they can be emotional in nature. V.K. was an overweight woman who said, "I hate looking at myself in the mirror every morning." She was put on Crab Apple amongst other things to cleanse her self-perception, which is one of ugliness and disgust. A few days into the essences, she called to complain that she loathed herself even more. When she was able to understand the cleansing process, she persisted with the doses and by the next day, the unsettling self-loathing went away. Another woman did not heed the advice. She was given Cherry Plum for her outbursts with her husband, which was disturbing the peace of the household. The night she started on the essences, she launched into a tirade at her husband. Alarmed, she poured the formula down the sink after deciding that it was really bad for her.

It helps to understand this cleansing process for what it is and not let fear get in the way of therapy. Such effects are a sure sign that you have the right essences; wrong essences could never produce a response. They are also always temporary and will only last as long as it takes to release all the negative vibrations targeted by the essences. One way to know for sure if you are experiencing a cleansing effect is to stop dosing and check if the symptoms go away. If they do, then you know that it is a result of therapy.

Some people may find it difficult to deal with this process. There are a few options here: (1) Stop taking the essences and the symptoms should go away. Try to identify the essence that is catalyzing the cleansing, and exclude it from your formula until a later time. This way, you can continue your work with the other essences. (2) You can add Rescue Remedy into your personal formula, or (3) alternate a dose of the formula with a dose of Rescue Remedy. Rescue Remedy can help to settle the sometimes difficult emotions that arise. (4) Reduce the frequency of dosing to a manageable level.

3. Positive Effects

A sense of well-being arrives when the person is relieved of their internal conflicts by the essences. The body is a reflection of the person's inner state, so the resulting inner peace and harmony may show itself physically. The face may turn clear and radiant, displaying perhaps a smiling and happier expression; the eyes become softer and brighter, or dreams can become more active and vivid. One client described how she found herself humming and singing, something she could not recall doing for years! Physical discomfort and illness can also improve or disappear.

4. Peeling Effect

A human being is a complex matrix of habits and patterns that are embedded in layers. A peeling phenomenon occurs with the use of the essences, and after some time – it could be weeks, months or years – a new set of layers may surface that cast light on deeper issues. As each layer is peeled off, another will surface. Depending on how many layers are in the personality outfit you wear, that is how much work you have to do. It varies widely among individuals. Those who consciously acknowledge and work on reducing their struggles will feel the impact of this work more quickly. Others who have not spent time investigating and learning what makes them tick will probably peel at a slower rate. The body also has its own timing – it will only allow the peeling to happen at a pace that you can handle and so again, there is no need to fear.

A Bach Consultation

The flower essences are primarily intended to be a means of self-help but it is not always easy to see oneself honestly and clearly to make the right choices. To address this, you can consult a Bach practitioner to jumpstart your process with the essences. There are two kinds of practitioners using Bach Flower Essences: those who have undergone training set out in the *Bach International Education Program* (BIEP) and those who have studied on their own and integrated the essences into their existing healing practice. The BIEP is offered in 20 countries worldwide. Successful completion of the program offers a person a place as a *Bach Foundation Registered Practitioner* (BFRP) on the International Register of Practitioners kept by The Edward Bach Foundation in the United Kingdom.

The role of a BFRP is more than just recommending essences. Using a simple consultation interview, the practitioner helps clients to define their goals for therapy, articulate their needs and put their problems into perspective. Because of their training, practitioners can also gain additional insights or detect under-currents of distress that would otherwise go unnoticed. The consultation process is both therapeutic and educational. Clients develop clarity and awareness of the conflicts within them and are empowered to work with the practitioner to arrive at an accurate selection of essences and to develop an individualized healing program.

My personal goal as a BFRP is three-fold. The short-term is to relieve the immediate suffering of the client; the medium to help the client stabilize by using the essences to peel off layers of unrest and conflict. The long-term goal is to help the client recover and empower their true essence. To accomplish this, we need to identify the core sensitivities that predispose the client to imbalance. With the right essences, the entire being can be maintained in a reasonable dynamic balance. Living from our essence becomes possible and we arrive at a true state of health. At each point of the journey, the choice to continue working or not always remains the client's.

Part III

Healing The Family

A personality without conflict
is immune to disease.

Dr Edward Bach
Heal Thyself

5

Helping Your Family

Bach Flower Essences are unrivalled in family therapy for a number of reasons. Firstly, you need not be equipped with theories of child psychology and development to use this modality. The Bach system offers a model based on human traits observable in any child or adult; traits so universal we can all recognize them with minimal training because they are part of our daily human experience. With some education and practice, a person can identify the appropriate essences for their situation and readily help themselves and others.

Secondly, the theories and models used in counseling appeal primarily to the conscious self, the part that exercises volition. For this reason, it is not always fully successful. Clients, who are psychotherapists and have worked extensively on themselves in their professional and personal development, acknowledge the inner struggles that still come up on old issues.

This shortcoming is particularly evident in cases of young children. Parents may send their 10-year-old child to a psychiatrist to deal with her panic attacks or temper outbursts. But how do you talk a child out of fear, anger or depression? Why should adults demand that children be able to choose and control how they think, feel and act when they themselves can fail so miserably at times? So many parents' frustration, irritation and despair come simply from setting unrealistic expectations. This work is different in that it directs therapy at the energetic source of the problem by releasing it with the essences.

Thirdly, this method acknowledges the interdependence of family dynamics on the energetic level, and offers a true path to dissolve the negative vibrations that hold a family at odds with each other. Its simplicity allows the entire family to use essences concurrently to bring about a painless dissolution of issues that prevent family members from enjoying mutually satisfying relationships.

Family therapy plays an especially crucial role when treating a child who lives in an extremely difficult situation at home, such as a hostile or an abusive one. We cannot help that child without taking care of the adults as well, because they have so much influence on him or her. Young children are immersed in the family environment for nearly 24 hours a day. In each moment, they are hearing, absorbing, understanding, perceiving, concluding all kinds of things and have little respite from that environment. Treating the child alone is not enough; the energetic influences from the environment continue to make inroads into the youngster. Thus it becomes very important in such cases for the adults to get involved in therapy, especially the parent who perceives the problem and the child perceived to have a problem.

The Loss Of Emotional Freedom

A lack of individuality (i.e. allowing interference with our individual unique nature) is of great importance in the genesis of disease. This interference begins early in life, and the after effects are extremely profound and, in most instances, stretch into the rest of one's life. So many problems we face as adults can be traced back to a conscious or unconscious decision made in the earlier period of our lives. My work with clients has impressed this deeply upon me and I have often wished I had gotten to the person while they were still a child and saved them years of suffering.

Dr Bach used the term 'moulding' to describe the family's interference with a child's natural state. Family dynamics are exceptionally complex. In a family unit, there is intense interaction amongst a group of people. The intensity is greatest immediately after birth and decreases as soon as the child grows and moves into expanded circles of influence. For most of us, the most intense and profound interaction would be with our mothers, albeit there are instances when children grow up with a single father, grandparents, relatives such as aunts and uncles or, in some cases, adopted, fostered or raised in orphanages.

In each moment of interaction, something very profound happens for the child. The child draws conclusions about the adult, experiences him or her in a certain way, feels for and develops an attitude about that person. All these experiences – whether it is a belief about the mother, a conclusion about oneself, or an experience of an emotion, a perception about life in general – are energy forms. They are energy forms that become lodged in our energy body. They remain even after the experience is over and will not go away until we actually release their vibrations from our system. Over time, you can imagine the multitude of impressions created with each adult. For every person involved, there is a specific set remaining with the child. On top of these, the child also layers on their decisions on how to respond to each person and in each situation.

You can now begin to understand why so few of us possess the emotional freedom to help another member of the family. Each time we are in their presence, this storehouse of impressions is activated and colors our experience and therefore reaction to them. We are trapped by past emotional imprints, bound by old beliefs and chained to previous perceptions of the other. It is no wonder that when it comes to helping family, we often get ourselves into a sticky tangle and tie ourselves into knots. Despite our good intentions, frustration, anger and discouragement run high whenever we try to pull someone out of a rut.

In this state, you cannot provide a safe and nurturing environment for another to address their problems. Your past issues with the person have reared their ugly heads and become a stumbling block to your aid. No one responds well to a helper who despises, disparages or scolds them. Such behavior only turns them off to your good intent and the situation, instead of improving, may degenerate further. If you find yourself in this dilemma, the best option is to use the essences to achieve some degree of emotional balance and mental clarity. It helps to do this before and during your efforts to be of service. Of course, it may take a while to rebalance yourself from years of unhealthy habits, and you may find that even after much work, you are still not the most effective candidate to go to someone's aid. It takes humility and love to accept this, and allow others to step in at this point.

The following sections deal with some very unconscious assumptions and behavior we exhibit when we try to help others. It pays to examine and understand them carefully. If we are to be true to our intention to help others, then whatever wrong views and unconstructive contributions we bring into the situation need to be abandoned to facilitate that process.

Check Your Motivation

It is tempting to make use of the essences to 'correct' the people who are close to us. Inevitably at every talk, some members of the audience become excited at the thought of slipping essences to their spouses, children or other family members. Certain personality types have a greater inclination to pursue and justify this, especially those in the Overcare category. **Chicory** individuals, for example, cannot restrain themselves from interfering and taking care of others regardless of whether their help is sought or not. The compelling perception that drives them is that they know best for those they love, and so hold the key to all solutions. They give no freedom for others to fail and fall, to make mistakes, or the space to work out their own choices and difficulties. Without them, the other would suffer collapse and fall apart. Unfortunately, this persistent interference only weakens those around them and wears out the Chicory person who is trying to hold up everyone. This trait is the classic cause of co-dependency.

The **Beech** personality is blinded by a veil of faults and flaws, which is projected onto everyone and everything around them. This critical and judgmental state makes it impossible for the person to be satisfied and to take delight in others. It sees little or no goodness in them. In their desire to eliminate this, the Beech will try to set things right. Why is Beech in the category of overcaring for others when their minds are so negative? Because they have learned to care by focusing on what's wrong in others and by reminding and correcting their faults as much as they can. In their own minds, they believe themselves to be making things better. There are others of course. Both **Vervain** and **Vine** types are insistent personalities: the Vervain through reasoning, persuasion, argument and anger as a last resort and the Vine through downright insistence and bullying.

When you catch yourself doing this, it may be wise to take a few moments to adjust your motivation. If you want to introduce essences to someone, do it out of love and not for your own convenience. Be aware that fixing others to alleviate one's own irritation and distress is a self-cherishing act no matter how altruistic we may think we are. Although no one can stop you from carrying on, it is certain that an improper motivation would make you an unhelpful agent in someone's healing process simply because your needs are on the agenda rather than theirs. No matter how much we are in denial of this, our body emanates our intentions and causes others to doubt and distrust us. Right from the beginning, we are doomed to fail. Indeed, if we cannot be dispassionate enough, it would be wiser and more effective to invite a third party to deliver the required assistance and support.

Wherever possible, it is better for therapy in the family to become a conscious process than to turn it into an underground mission. With a spouse or older children, I suggest that there be a discussion and an agreement first. If they have no wish to take the essences, just keep working on yourself. Sometimes, the changes in you will inspire them to do something about themselves. At other times, you will find that what you found so irritating about the other person actually disappears when you heal your own mental and emotional perception of things.

There are, of course, circumstances that permit us to decide and prepare essences for others without their consent. Young children who are facing mental-emotional challenges need help from the adults. In elderly cases where the individual no longer has the faculty to make their own decisions, someone who is very ill or in an emergency situation, compassion demands that we take action to relieve the other's suffering. One mother had to watch as her son suffered from a drug addiction. She took it upon herself to slip essences into his food, drink, anything that he put into his mouth. One day, the son caught her in the act and said: "Whatever you are doing, just keep on doing it." He had obviously experienced the benefits and appreciated his mother's intention. The bottomline is this: if love and kindness are in charge of the decision, then allow yourself to do the best for the other.

The Self-Centered Approach

Why do we suffer when we try to help another? In the process of helping, we sometimes watch ourselves move through a spectrum of emotions. Intentions can initially be kind and caring, but when faced with obstacles, opposition or objection, we move into impatience and frustration, which can then progress to anger, resentment and hostility. Finally, as futility sets in, we descend into helplessness and hopelessness. We blame the person(s) we are helping for the trauma we have to go through in order to help them, and justify giving up. We end up getting all entangled and knotted up, and wish we had never gotten involved in the first place. A positive choice turns into regret, even damaging relationships. This is how we reason ourselves into disregarding future impulses of kindness and compassion.

There are many reasons why things can go wrong. Perhaps we do not have the right skills or information; wrong diagnosis of the problem also leads to ineffective solutions. Oftentimes it is because we take every response to our help too personally; everything is about us. When a **Vervain** or **Vine** does not follow our advice, it is because they have no respect for us. When a **Willow** blames us instead of thanking us, we are hurt and abandon them. When a **Scleranthus** is still unable to decide and act after hours of counseling, we condemn them for wasting our time. When a **Chestnut Bud** keeps making the same mistake, we think they are intentionally trying to annoy us. Of course these characters will behave the way they do; these are their traits and are to be expected. Insisting on their ways, the Vine is obstinate and the Vervain rebels; the Willow begrudges, the Scleranthus is indecisive and the Chestnut Bud does not learn from their mistakes. Their response to our help is *not* about us; it is about them and the very thing for which they need help. To simply have this single understanding, one can immediately disengage from the negativity, stay clear of the reactions and focus on finding creative ways to resolve the issue at hand.

Most of us, however, do not possess such a magnanimous view. Instead, we take everything personally and we become part of the problem. This self-referential approach takes attention away from the object of our compassion to our own personal issues. We forget about the other and begin to focus on our negativity that has been activated, of course always perceiving and blaming the other person as the cause. There is tremendous vanity and, at the same time, suffering in this way of perceiving things. Herein lies the biggest source of complication when we are trying to help others.

❀ Effective Helping

Effective helping grows out of a genuine concern for others and some common sense practices. We don't necessarily have to attend classes to learn these; they are natural skills that come by with some forethought and compassion.

A good working alliance between helper and helpee is at the core of successful helping and at the center of this is **acceptance**. One deeply effective way of cultivating acceptance is to develop a proper understanding of the helpee's situation and reality. Every individual is fundamentally whole and sound. Whatever habitual patterns and behavior they display are the very illnesses to be treated. *They are not their problems, their negative emotions or their destructive habits.* We can dislike the energetic patterns that destroy happiness, but we do not have to simultaneously reject the individual because of our own confusion. Holding others in this way – focusing on their fundamental goodness – is the best way to practice acceptance. It arises out of wisdom, not ruled by politically, spiritually or principly correct responses. Helping others because we *should, must, have* or *ought to* is limiting by its very nature. No matter how much we try to put on the 'correct' and 'dutiful' compassionate act, our objections to the other person are communicated energetically nonetheless. We emanate criticism, resentment, aversion, scorn and intolerance incongruent with our spoken intentions. Our body language cannot lie; therefore from the beginning, honesty, sincerity and authenticity are crucial building blocks of a good rapport with someone we want to help.

Communication provides the information to base your selection of essences. Therefore the ability to allow the helpee to talk, clarify and define their issues is a useful one. Active and responsive listening is an art; a powerful tool to acknowledge, validate and accept someone when used skillfully. When we listen well, we hear beyond the words and through the body. Much can be communicated and learned in this fashion, and one can be like a detective picking up clues and a trail that would have otherwise been overlooked. There were many instances in my own practice where the need for essences were identified not so much from what the client said, but how they said it and what they chose or neglected to say.

Some personality types would obviously encounter difficulties with listening. It is not the **Vine's** habit to listen to others. They are the leaders who take charge. So certain are their assessment and solutions that they often override others' input to get their way. The **Impatiens** is eager for action, so would see talking and listening as a waste of time. The **Heather** will turn everyone's calamity into a talking point for their own cause. They cannot hear because they are busy talking about themselves. It can be equally difficult to communicate with a **Vervain**. This type is overly attached to their views and opinions, tend to insist, persuade and argue for others to come round to their stance. The **Agrimony**, with a habit of denial, finds it a challenge to face their issues. Therefore listening and acknowledging another's distress would unlikely be something they desire to do even when necessary. Uncomfortable with displays of emotions, they do not know what to do and may walk away. Some can even go so far as to ignore or pretend the problem is not there. It would be hard for this parent type to sit down with a child to discuss problems or conflicts, and so help cannot even begin.

Other avenues of information are readily available in a home setting. Daily observations and experiences of the family member concerned are equally valuable in the overall assessment.

Empathy is cultivated by putting ourselves in the other's shoes. This is the best technique to stay present to the other. When we are helping someone, it is not about us, it is about them. In class, my students commonly project problems when trying to work out an essence selection. Reading through a case study, they decide how they would feel under those circumstances and end up recommending essences for themselves. They fail to attend to the actual complaints presented and would miss some of the essences indicated. This is a widespread phenomenon and the cause of many failures in the delivery of assistance.

Self-awareness and **personal responsibility** requires a degree of courage and training but ensures a means of separating our own issues from those of the person we are helping. When negative emotions and attitudes come up in us, we have to bear responsibility for them. Take for example a woman who was extremely suspicious of her husband in his relationship with female colleagues. Whichever way she turned, her friends only helped to stoke the fire of jealousy and suspicion further. They were angry and upset with her husband, taught her ways to keep him in check and how to punish him. Her problem became their problem. These well-intentioned women gave advice tainted by their own prejudices and could not provide impartial assistance to the couple. Finally, this woman turned to the essences and within a week, this particular marital problem happily disappeared.

Another example is the **Rock Water** type who lives such an idealized life that they have lost touch with their own and others' reality. A great deal of arrogance exists in the Rock Water who hands down the 'shoulds' and 'should nots', 'musts' and 'must nots'. This type often lectures those who seek their help, which can add on to the suffering of someone already troubled. It is wise and compassionate to acknowledge our own failings and weaknesses, to understand our humanness so that when we have the good fortune to help another, we do not do so from a high place or for the purpose of elevating ourselves.

How we are is how we help. If we were a **Gentian** easily disheartened and lacking faith in the outcome of our efforts, we carry that pessimism into the situation. We help unconsciously expecting things not to work out, or for the person not to change. If we were resentful like a **Willow**, then we would resent those who come to us for help. What one person sees as a delightful opportunity to be of service turns into a curse and burden to a Willow. A **Water Violet** withdraws because they do not want to be troubled and involved. A **Wild Rose** typically advises acceptance and resignation because that is their own mode of operation. The uncertainty of the **Scleranthus** and **Cerato** makes it impossible for them to give any advice or take any action. They themselves do not know what to do. Every one of us can only benefit at the level to which we are healed of these habits ourselves. The higher our self-awareness and understanding, the greater the benefits we offer. Since the elements of effective helping also increase automatically, our help also flows more effortlessly.

We must also not forget that we can only help those who want to help themselves. When there is a match between the helpee's and helper's intention, something magical happens. This has repeated itself so evidently in my work. Clients with a high level of desire to get well naturally make the best healers. They are focused on their goals, willing to do whatever it takes and willing to work with the practitioner. Those with unconscious agendas take a longer time and have a shaky commitment to therapy. Even though I may put out my best effort and take away their imaginary conditions for healing, in the end it is their intention that does not hold up strong and long enough. As the saying goes, "You can take the horse to the water, but you cannot make it drink."

Even then, this is not synonymous with giving up on the individual. Every one of us has a way of working out our struggles and evolving. In our very limited concept of time and space, we are unable to accept this and make our personal struggle with this an unnecessary component of the problem. It does take a great deal of patience and a great deal of love and, in the end, it is patience and love that heals more than anything we can do.

Overview Of Section

The following three chapters deal with various areas of family life:

- ### Resolving Family Issues

Examines some challenges commonly faced by families, and how to use the essences to ease and dissolve them.

- ### Growing Up As A Parent

Helps parents to understand their individual parenting stress, conflicts and limitations, and how to use the essences to eliminate them.

- ### Nurturing Your Child

Describes the challenges of growing up, and how parents can apply the essences to help their children retain their natural essence, thus empowering them to health and to life.

The treatment of topics in these chapters is by no means complete. The multitudes and variations of family dynamics can never be fully covered in a simple book like this, and it is not the author's purpose to do so. It is written with the hope, however, that sufficient information and illustrations are provided to help readers make the connection between the essences and family life, and inspire them to action. With a proper understanding, you can learn to free your families from much unnecessary suffering by exploring and reaping the benefits offered by the 38 Bach flowers.

6

Resolving Family Issues

A good friend asked, "Why should parents take the essences if it is the child who has the problem?" Indeed, many parents who seek my help come precisely with that attitude. The problem is with the child; the problem is separate from me. It is the child who needs help. This attitude brings to question a number of fundamental assumptions that we have taken for granted.

Unthinkingly, we view our perception and experience of a person, an event or problem as definitive. In actuality, there are multiple perspectives. If the child is inherently bad, then he or she should upset everyone in the same way. But it is quite obvious in our experience that this is not always so. One child's habit can trigger off an adult's wrath, cheer up another and receive a shrug from the next. Our perceptions and experiences are obviously highly dependent on something other than the child – *our own personality traits, attitudes and habitual emotions.* How we perceive things determines how we respond and how we respond determines how we suffer or not suffer. On good days, we are more likely to brush aside something that normally irritates us; but when we are in a bad mood, the smallest thing can trigger off a stream of harsh speech, frustration, criticism or depression.

We bring into each moment of interaction so much of our past history of experiences, which colors our perception and obscures us to the moment. Unless we are mentally clear and emotionally poised, we are unable to assess a situation accurately. This is important to understand in family dynamics, which is highly interdependent in nature. Problems in interactions are generated simultaneously and so to resolve them, the best approach is to dissolve them simultaneously too.

For this reason, I often encourage the parent(s) to join their child in therapy, to help them consider their own attitudes and projections that could contribute to the issues. It is of course ideal to have everyone in the family using the essences, but this is difficult to come by. The more important partner for the child in therapy is the parent who perceives him or her to have or to be a problem. When both parent and child work together, the dynamics can shift rapidly as they both reach for balance. Of course, not everyone takes this advice. Some parents insist on being separate, but there are also others whose love gives them the courage to examine themselves. Mothers are likely to take this option and they are often pleasantly surprised by the result.

In this chapter, we explore some issues and situations that a family has to face, either as individuals or as a group. The list is limited both in the problems discussed as well as the essences that can apply. They are only a handful to illustrate the relevance of the flower essences to understand and heal family dynamics.

✿ Communication

If you look at a **Water Violet** plant in its habitat, you can get an idea of the state of mind that its flowers treat. A Water Violet grows well out in the middle of ponds and streams, difficult to reach. Each plant holds up a solitary flower stem, rising tall, erect and delicate from the surface of the water with the flowers clustered at its pinnacle. This personality type is equally comfortable in their solitude. Quiet and self-reliant, they prefer their own company and so spend a fair amount of time alone.

They are unobtrusive people who keep to themselves and leave others alone. A Water Violet therefore has difficulty easing into social interaction. It does not matter if it is with a group of colleagues at work or with family members and relatives. Highly selective in the type of people they allow into their lives, they prefer one-to-one interaction with other quiet types. They are economical and functional in their speech, and a minimalist in conversations. They usually speak just enough and when spoken to.

In less familiar and larger social settings, their solitary nature becomes especially evident to them. Many Water Violet types describe their situations with uncannily similar words: "I feel like a bystander in life, an observer but not a participant." "I feel even more alone in crowds than when I am by myself."

You can see how easily a Water Violet can become distant from the spouse or children. One father's complaint was that he felt increasingly left out of the family. His children and wife were becoming closer as the children grew older, but he was unable to bridge the widening gap between him and them. His growing teenage daughters saw him as aloof and unapproachable and had moved away from him, which brought much pain. His Water Violet trait was a personal habit, compounded by the fact that he traveled and worked alone for long periods of time.

Between husband and wife, this Water Violet coolness and distance was easily mistaken as a reflection of the partner's undesirability, a lack of love and interest. Left uncorrected, the couple drifted apart over time never really understanding why. In the above case, the wife was an **Aspen** type, nervous and anxious of things unknown. Unable to comprehend that she did not cause her husband's response and that he had brought this trait into the marriage, she became anxious around him, second-guessing his silence and aloofness. Is he unhappy with me? Is his silence disapproval? Was it something I had done wrong? She never knew because he never communicated, and she never asked because she was afraid. To avoid this anxiety around him, she moved away and so personal communication ceased between husband and wife; the only time they spoke was when it concerned the children.

A child would find it challenging to communicate with a Water Violet parent. It is hard to engage them in conversation, to expect full participation in their daily affairs or a display of warmth and affection. Children do not easily understand such behavior, and can perceive and react to it in a multitude of ways: "My father (or mother) is not interested in me; he (or she) doesn't love me." "There is something wrong with me, which is why nobody talks to me," or "It is not okay to be lively, exuberant and expressive." Silence can become a norm. A lack of communication, or no communication, can distance members of the family and turn them into strangers under the same roof. Children can become totally withdrawn. The lonely circumstances in which an only child grows up can also predispose them to the Water Violet trait.

The Water Violet flower helps a person to break free of this misconception of separateness and dissolves the barrier and awkwardness between them and others. It does not take away their quiet, peaceful nature but provides a social ease that can alleviate much of the loneliness they often experience over time. The essence acts like a social lubricant, allowing this personality type to open up, connect and enjoy the company of others.

A **Heather** personality is the reverse of the Water Violet. They talk easily and much but still have a communication problem. In a severely out-of-balance state, the Heather talks incessantly and indiscriminately about anything as long as it is about them. It could be their hairstyle, dentures, bowel movement; it could be their children, garden, pets or their shoes and closet. Conversations tend to be monologues and are not meant to be communicative, but to assuage their loneliness and fear of being alone. Heather spouses are demanding and needy of attention for that reason. The individual can be so severely self-obsessed as to become narcissistic, where the relationship is all about them and no one else.

Out of habitual self-absorption, the Heather parent talks on and on about themselves even when they are with their children. One client in her fifties described how her mother would download her marital problems onto her, including some aspects of the marriage that were totally inappropriate to discuss with a child. Conversations were seldom focused on the young girl:

what was going on in her life, how she was doing in school. A complex mixture of beliefs was built up around this. She felt guilty because she could not do anything to help her mother. She felt burdened, heavy with the problems of the adults. She also felt insignificant, unimportant and ignored. These challenges were to plague the entirety of her adult life.

Similarly, we may find children who grow up in lonely environments and who compensate by over-engaging socially. They are the talkative little ones who chatter on about nothing and everything. Their ME, ME, ME syndrome makes it difficult for other children and even adults to enjoy them. One client, who had to endure a lonely childhood because of a sick mother, grew up talking to himself. In his forties, he was still talking aloud to himself at home. Extremely afraid of being alone, he latches on to people in social gatherings, but this neediness simply drives them away and has badly affected his chances of a serious relationship. He also had to endure being labeled 'weird' for his strange behavior.

Lopsided, self-centered conversations hold little attraction for most people. Many avoid or move away from Heather types, making them feel even lonelier. The Heather essence helps to take the person's mind off themselves, so they can have the space to see, hear and be present to others and to cultivate mutually fulfilling and satisfying connections. The Heather state is quite difficult to see in ourselves, perhaps because it is rather unpleasant to admit to such self-obsession. However, we need not be excessively talkative to qualify for this essence. Whenever we are too preoccupied and engrossed with ourselves – on the good or the bad – we can use some Heather to restore our balance.

In the case of an **Agrimony**, the problem is a lack of authentic communication. The Agrimony type is a joker and clown. They wear a cheerful face, make light of things and are seldom serious. One never knows how the Agrimony actually feels, what they really want or need. They can be a bit of a Jekyll and Hyde: the father who is a model of a man outside the family, a wonderful host to friends and then, in the safe environment of home, abuses the family. Or the mother who charms everyone in the social circle and then hides in the room drinking from a bottle of alcohol.

The humor and charm of an Agrimony hides a deep-seated distress. Such persons have difficulty acknowledging, understanding and working with their inner experiences. They may be troubled, tormented, restless and worrying but they intensely dislike and do not know how to deal with inner conflicts and negative emotions. They want peace internally and externally, and the price they are willing to pay is to keep up a pretense. They can often turn to external substances such as drugs, alcohol or food to numb and avoid their distress.

It can be infuriating when the situation requires some serious action and you have a spouse who takes everything lightly. That can be a source of bickering. One male client made some bad choices and lost a great deal of his company's money, was laid off and lived in fear of legal prosecution. The very distraught wife blamed him for destroying everything they had and ruining the family. She found his ability to joke about the situation not only inappropriate but infuriating. His smiling and breezy manner only drove her through the roof. In session, the man expressed deep remorse and had tears in his eyes. He had always ignored things, tried to make everyone happy and joked to be a nice guy. Now he could no longer hold back his emotions: he wanted to break down and cry, and was experiencing uncontrollable angry episodes where he would hit out at things. He was afraid to allow these emotions in public, and for this reason sought help. For him, an additional essence **Cherry Plum** became necessary to treat his fear of losing control. The wife who could not comprehend his bizarre behavior continued to misunderstand and blame him. She felt justified in her anger and so forfeited the opportunity to deal with her own issues.

You can also have an Agrimony child who makes light of what the parents say, again giving rise to conflicts. If the parents take it personally, as an act of insolence and disrespect, of course they will be upset and irritated. However, with a little spaciousness of mind, they can entertain another possibility. The problem is not about them; it is about the child. Their child's happy face and light-hearted attitude could indicate an Agrimony pattern of denial and suppression, an inability to address the inner going-ons that generate unseen distress and torment. As parents, if they are able to assess the situation properly instead of becoming personal about it, they would then see the need for this essence to help him or her.

Absenteeism

The trademark of a **Vervain** is over-effort. In daily life, this translates into an overabundance of energy and enthusiasm, over-achieving and excessively strong attachment to personal views, beliefs and principles. When the parent is an over-achiever at work, they will be away from home most of the time. This is the workaholic parent who takes on extra work voluntarily and one project after another. Adult Vervains are valued for their drive and ability to accomplish a lot. Their only downfall is that they do not know how to stop before they burn up all their energy.

They are intense individuals – intense in their speech, in their emotions, intense in their work and play. Another obvious trait about a Vervain is how passionate and attached they are to their views of right and wrong, which they feel necessary to impose on others. Highly principled individuals, they champion the underdogs, spending a great deal of time and effort to right the social and moral injustices of the world. What upsets the balance of a Vervain is a perceived injustice, and much anger and outrage can result. At home, a child's retort to a Vervain parent could bring on the famous "How dare you speak to me like that!"

One client in his thirties had this to say about his mother: "My mother was never around when I was young. She was in this club and this society and president of that organization. She was fighting all these battles for people in the world but she was never around for the family." This is how an overly active Vervain parent or parents can easily be drawn away from the home and become physically absent while their children are growing up.

The Vervain child is equally energetic and hyperactive. They cannot keep still and need to move from one activity to another. At play, these children put their bodies to maximum use and do not stop till they collapse from exhaustion. In the classroom, they can have difficulty paying attention, be rebellious and defiant against authority and play truant from school. Or they are the students *par excellence* who excel in academics and everything else. Their imbalance is an over-abundance of energy inside them, which they try to expend by doing a great deal. Like the adult version, the children are equally intense in every way. Parents can find it difficult to discipline their Vervain children – the little Vervain can be as adamant about their rights as their Vervain parent – or to keep up with their boundless energy.

The flower essence helps to rebalance the energy use of Vervains, so that they do not expend energy wantonly. When they come into balance, they are able to hold and direct their energy resources in the way they want, instead of being driven and controlled by them. Another positive effect of this essence is to loosen the attachment to one's views and the need to be right. Arguments are generated from Vervain imbalances, when individuals in relationships feel strongly about their point of view and need to justify, argue and insist on being right. Since we have all experienced this at one time or another, we therefore do not need to be Vervain types to use this essence.

The **Clematis** parent is outwardly passive but mentally active. Typical words to describe this type are spacey, dreamy and drowsy. They are preoccupied with their own imaginary world, wrapped up in their thoughts. If they are unhappy or in conflict, the tendency is to escape into a make-belief world to conjure up images and fantasies of better times. Because they are highly imaginative, they have many good ideas but do not possess the physical presence to do the necessary work to manifest them. They usually lack awareness of their environment and find it hard to give full attention to the people in their lives. To a child, a Clematis parent can be hard to reach and engage. They are physically present but emotionally absent, which can lead to both physical and emotional neglect.

One woman described how she sat in front of the TV to sort out the family photo albums. One hour later, she woke up from her reverie, sitting there with photo albums still undone and the TV still on. Where had she been all this time? She had spaced out completely for a full hour! Another young college student described how he walked all the way to a lecture hall only to remember it was the wrong one when he reached there.

You can recognize the same sleepy, dreamy state in a child with a Clematis tendency. This is the child who stares wide-eyed at the TV screen, totally immobile. It is quite obvious they are not engaged in the program as their eyes are not following the happenings on the screen. In the classroom, they daydream and fail to pay attention and may be struggling with grades. You will find clues to a Clematis child in the way they entertain themselves with make-belief games, whether it is a little girl engrossed in playing doll or a young boy in sci-fi fantasy. Because they have little awareness of the external environment, they may also be clumsy, forgetful and accident prone.

Many Clematis actually enjoy the dreamy state that preoccupies them. In that imaginary world, they can conjure up whatever makes them happy; in reality, they do not have such a choice. Therefore it can be and often is a way to escape from the drudgery, difficulties or unhappiness in their present circumstances. The Clematis flower helps to ground the individual in their physical body and to rebalance their mental and physical being. They become more present to their surroundings, are able to interact appropriately and translate their imaginings into creative forms. For the parent, this means being aware of and being available to their children and for the children, it means paying attention to the world around them and being able to learn and grow with it.

The **Mustard** essence is for depression. This is a type of depression that descends and lifts without any known reason. For someone who needs Mustard, melancholy and gloom is the state of mind and the most puzzling part of it is that it cannot be attributed to any circumstances in their lives. Dark moods engulf them, making it hard to live each day with purpose and joy. When the depression is gripping, it paralyzes the person so they cannot work, cannot eat, cannot sleep or sleep all the time. Sadness and helplessness can overwhelm and debilitate them. They lose interest in things and people around them, cannot focus or concentrate and may have recurring thoughts about suicide and death. In severe cases, they cannot even get up to wash their face or feed themselves. One woman described her experiences: "I go to bed at 5pm so I would not hurt myself. I felt a lot of anger and aggression. It is as if someone came and took all my power away."

The effects of depression are both devastating and heartbreaking for family members. Any child will find it difficult to grow up in an environment without laughter, pleasure and joy. Prolonged gloom affects everyone adversely. If it is the parent who suffers from crippling depression, not only are they physically and emotionally unavailable for the child but the child may well end up being the caretaker of the parent. She or he becomes a parent for the parent who has become their child, an overwhelming responsibility that weighs heavy on little shoulders. To watch a parent suffer from depression – the inconsistent behavior, the unexpected tears, the inability to function and terrible unhappiness – is confusing for one so young. These children have to grow up very quickly in order to cope with the family situation. They can feel overwhelmed (**Elm**), guilty and responsible (**Pine**), and helpless and hopeless (**Gorse**). Postpartum depression is another puzzling phenomenon that affects some women after childbirth. It can be accompanied by irrational thoughts to harm the newborn, a **Cherry Plum** state. One mother questioned, "How can a mother feel depressed and anxious and not be happy with such a beautiful baby?" Yet the depression was a reality for her.

Mustard helps to lift the depression, so the person can reconnect with their *joie de vivre*. In this state, they are better able to enjoy their own and the lives of loved ones. Other essences that can assist in the symptoms that arise are **Cherry Plum** for suicidal thoughts, **Gorse** for the helplessness and hopelessness, **Sweet Chestnut** if there is deep anguish and despair. Depression still carries its stigma and the behavior of depressed people is still considered by some to be self-indulgent, self-pitying and plain selfish. Such views alienate and isolate those who really need our help, and make **Water Violet** necessary to relieve the terrible loneliness that comes about.

Abuse

Domestic violence has become an increasingly common occurrence in the household. Abuse can happen to spouses, children and the elderly. The **Cherry Plum**, with a highly explosive and volatile personality, has a tendency to lose control of themselves. We see this in men who batter their wives and children or hurl verbal abuses at them, or mothers who are equally capable of doing the same to their young ones. These individuals suffer from an inability to control and contain themselves. Some have no wish to do what they know to be wrong but the impulse to hit out overwhelms them. There are others who are so far gone in this direction that the thought to hold back does not even occur to them. They are highly reactive and hot-headed. The flower essence relieves the fear of loss of control or the actual loss of control.

Sometimes the loss of control comes because the abuser is under the influence of alcohol. For such cases, the emotional cause for their addiction must be treated as well for it is the alcohol that removes their inhibitions and self-control. **Vine** is another category who would likely bully their way through differences and conflicts. They use coercion and force to quell opposition. Taking the Vine essence helps to soften the tendency to dominate and overpower others by will. The abuser can also be afflicted by the **Holly** cold-hearted hatred and malice that gives them delight in hurting their victims.

Centaury women who have low self-worth and an inability to assert themselves suffer most in an abusive relationship. They do not feel strong enough to stand up for themselves, and succumb in part to appease and in part from fear. Their defense is to endure and absorb the insults and injury inflicted upon them until they cannot bear it anymore. This pattern can be perpetuated by an age-old belief, handed down from one generation of women to another, that this is the virtue and role of a woman. Foolish as it sounds, even educated women can still subscribe to and suffer from this unconscious belief to some extent.

One client found herself trapped in three consecutive abusive relationships. In the first, her husband arranged for her to go through three plastic surgeries to modify her body to his liking. Because of her severe Centaury imbalance, it never occurred to her that she had a right to say no. Instead, she only pleaded to be spared but without success. After the surgeries, she became physically ill for years. With an intense desire to be well, she took the essences with great diligence and frequency. The Centaury essence transformed this woman within a couple of months. She has reached a point in her healing where she wants to leave the current relationship, another abusive one. This is a major triumph for her – she is leaving not because she cannot bear any more abuse but because she wants a better life for herself. The Centaury essence has this empowering effect on the mind that feels weak and powerless. A **Vervain** woman would react very differently to abuse. She would retaliate and fight for her rights. This, of course, often intensifies the quarrels and fights, making it much harder for the young witnesses because there are now two persons instead of one abusing each other.

Children who grow up in an abusive environment live in fear – the fear of the next shouting match, the next fight between mom and dad, or the next attack on them. **Rock Rose** is useful for the panic and terror that grips them. They also develop the **Aspen** type of fear, an uneasy apprehension about what is to come. This fear puts a child on edge all the time, walking on eggshell in the house, wary and uncertain of what to expect the next moment. Left untreated, the child grows up with this underlying anxiety and apprehension. As adults, this Aspen fear will be triggered easily by any kind of uncertainty and for them, will be their main source of stress. E.M., a woman in her forties, grew up in a violent and tumultuous environment. At home, she had to cope with her mother's and her own abuse. Outside, violence, fighting and danger everywhere plagued her birth country. The impact of a terrifying and disruptive childhood persists to this day in her fearful and anxious nature. Now a mother herself, she projects this anxiety onto her own little girl and the cycle will likely continue until and unless her own childhood fear is released.

The child can also develop a **Red Chestnut** type of fear, fearing for the welfare of the spouse under attack and the safety of siblings. The same can be true of the abused spouse who can just as easily develop the Aspen and Red Chestnut fears, this time fearing for the children's welfare and safety. The **Holly** state is another common one in the abused who develops hatred, malice and a vengeful attitude towards their abuser. For others, a **Willow** resentment against the perpetrator poisons their lives and chances for happiness for a very long time.

Jealousy And Rivalry

Sibling rivalry can happen when an older child has difficulty adjusting to the arrival of a new one. Until then, as the only child, they are used to being the sole focus of attention of the parents, and probably everyone else as well. Sharing – whether it is affection, attention, space and toys – can be especially difficult for such children.

The essence **Holly** alleviates the vexations of jealousy: the hatred, the malice and desire to hurt and harm the other's happiness. Other applicable essences are **Chicory** for the territorial and possessive behavior and **Walnut** to stabilize the siblings involved. The latter can help an older child adjust to life with another sister or brother and protect the younger one from the sibling's negative energy. Sometimes the rivalry is not between siblings. It may be the father, jealous of the attention the infant is receiving from his wife, who needs help.

Nine-year-old R.I. was brought to me for a consultation by his mother. She was concerned by his menacing hostility towards his sisters, especially the latest addition, a 6-month-old girl. The mother worried that one day, he would really hurt them very badly. He complained that the mother did not pay him enough attention and, in session, admitted to feeling neglected and that nobody cared. Everyday was a fighting match between mother and son and when pushed too hard, he threatened suicide.

He was given the essences **Holly** for the malice and jealousy, **Chicory** for possessiveness, **Vervain** and **Vine** for his extremely rebellious and strong-willed traits, and **Cherry Plum** for the loss of control. As the eldest and the only boy, **Walnut** was given to help him adjust to life with his younger sisters and also to protect from his mother's negative emotions and intolerance towards him. He responded so well to the essences that in a week, the mother called to say that she could not recognize her own child!

This is an extreme case of course, but the childish malice is obvious and needs to be addressed before it leads to any misadventure. Fighting siblings can get some help with **Vine** if one or both are domineering, **Cherry Plum** for the emotional and physical loss of control, and **Centaury** to provide some added strength to the weaker one.

For some, sibling rivalry continues into teenage years and adulthood. They compete ferociously, trying to outdo each other, to vie for attention and to become the favorite child. Favoritism is a most harmful practice from parents. The less favored ones start to develop an inferiority complex (**Larch**), become bitter and resentful (**Willow**), or turn defiant and strong-willed in righting the injustice they have suffered, in which case they will need help with **Vervain**.

Then of course, there is the hatred, jealousy and suspicion between spouses. One young woman spoke about the cold war that went on between her parents for years, initiated by her mother. The mother would cook for the family but refused to allow the father to eat with them. At mealtimes, he had to make his way out of the door to find food for himself. This continued to the day he died. This type of **Holly** spousal treatment destroys a child on the inside. They feel torn between parents, a **Scleranthus** state, and cannot enjoy the warmth and harmony so needed for them to grow up emotionally balanced and healthy.

Another client described how she grew up in an environment poisoned by her father's suspicious and jealous nature. He often accused his wife of being unfaithful to him and every quarrel centered round the wife's perceived infidelity. The conflict in the marriage was extremely disruptive and traumatic for the children who literally grew up in a war zone. Another man brought his wife to me because she was increasingly jealous of his interaction with every woman. Her suspicion kept her awake at night and triggered off many heated exchanges. **Holly** is useful whether the suspicion is valid or not. This state of mind is hateful, vengeful and malicious and is harmful to the person feeling that way. In that state of vexation, nothing can be resolved; only hurtful words and actions spoken and done in the heat of the moment that can damage a relationship for life.

Family Feuds

It is not only Romeo and Juliet who suffered so tragically from a family feud. When asked, many families would be able to provide similar feuding stories in their lineage. How often do we hear someone say, "I have not spoken to my father in the last 10 years"? "My aunt and uncle have cut off all connection in the last two decades after their fight over who would take care of my grandmother." "I cannot forgive my brothers for being leeches, bleeding off my money. I don't want to have anything to do with them anymore." In one case, not only did the client not talk to the father but all the siblings made it a point not to mention him in conversation throughout their adulthood. My client, the youngest, was turning 50 then and so you can imagine how long this had been going on.

The causes for family feuds can be trivial, and the parties involved may have long forgotten the reason why the feud began in the first place, yet the anger and resentment are held onto tenaciously through the years. **Willow** is the main culprit for such long-standing grudges. This type does not forget and forgive easily. They can stay bitter and resentful to the end of their lives. The resentment burns like embers and slowly eats away at the person's capacity to be happy. Over time, they can become hardened and withdraw from life resentfully. The **Vervain** anger can also sustain family feuds when an injustice is perceived to have been committed against the injured party. The **Holly** hatred arising from jealousy, suspicion, envy and malice is another source of fuel. Sometimes **Honeysuckle** is a useful addition to help these people shake off the ugly memories of the past. Those who bear grudges fail to understand that their anger and resentment cannot hurt anyone except themselves. While the other parties have moved on with their lives, they imprison themselves in an unhappy past by refusing to experience the grace of forgiving and letting go.

✿ Transitions

Walnut is the essence for change. It helps to protect the mind and stabilizes it during times of transition. Changes can come in many forms, beginning with newlyweds starting a life together. Newly married couples can find their love much challenged by extremely mundane affairs, as one old friend discovered. A few months after his wedding, he complained, "We cannot even agree on how the dishes should be washed!"

Beech can help to relieve the irritation and intolerance at little idiosyncrasies and habits each partner brings into their married life. **Walnut** aids adjustment to a new system in the household, quite different from the one they had been brought up with. Daughters-in-law and mothers-in-law, whether living apart or together, may also need a strong dose of both to avoid unpleasant clashes. **Chicory** should be added if there is possessiveness from one or both parties, and **Vervain** if anger and arguments arise because each is insisting on their opinions and ways in the household.

In the course of a family's history, there may well be many more expected or desired transitions – birth of a child, bringing a pet into the family, a child starting school, moving house, changing jobs or marriage partners, relocating to another country. In all instances, Walnut facilitates a smooth transition. When children leave home to pursue their studies, work or to start their own families, parents whose lives have been absorbed with their children can miss them sorely. Here, **Walnut** will help them adjust to the change and **Honeysuckle** to release their attachment to the past. The **Chicory** type wants and needs the children to stay close to them and will hurt most from the separation.

Retirement is another challenge for some senior parents. After a full and busy life, it can be hard to adjust to a life of leisure and truly relax and enjoy one's retirement. The combination of **Walnut** and **Honeysuckle** can be equally appropriate in this instance. Here the Honeysuckle tackles the problem of missing their work, colleagues or even the work place.

Unforeseen Circumstances

● **Financial Hardships** – With the current uncertain economic climate, a family may find its financial situation challenged by retrenchment or losses in business or investments. The resulting stress can be hard to bear for the breadwinner of the family. One client was near a nervous breakdown at work. Her husband had lost his job, and now she was afraid she was going to lose hers because of a mistake she had made at work. She could not sleep worrying about the problem all the time; she was fearful over the precarious financial situation, anxious over the uncertain future and reproaching herself endlessly for the mistake she had made. She was ready to snap. **Mimulus** (for the fear of not having enough money), **Aspen** (for the anxiety over uncertainty of her job), **White Chestnut** (for the continuous worries), **Pine** (to relieve the self-reproach and blame) and **Cherry Plum** (for the severe mental strain) were indicated for this case.

Gentian is useful for those who are unsuccessful in one job application after another. It eliminates discouragement and lack of faith in a positive outcome from their efforts. However, some may be worn out faster than others and disappointment can quickly turn into hopelessness and despair, which can be eliminated by **Gorse**. In extreme financial loss, the shock and anguish can be tremendous and sometimes long lasting. **Star of Bethlehem** addresses the trauma and **Sweet Chestnut** for the agonizing despair. A few individuals may not be able to get over the loss and begin to entertain suicidal thoughts. It is of utmost importance to take care of this unbalanced state immediately with **Cherry Plum** so the thoughts do not spin out of control and turn into unfortunate action. Cherry Plum helps to return the mind its calm and rationale.

• **Separation or Divorce** – At times, the relationship between couples takes a downward spiral and goes on a course of no return. Often, it is because the couple has not addressed problems as they arise and only took action when the situation has escalated to a state they can no longer ignore. Men and women invest a great deal into a marriage, so of course a separation or divorce would be traumatic for them, and even more so to the children. **Star of Bethlehem** aids in the grieving process. For the child, it is the loss of the family as he or she knew it; for the adults, it is the grief and heartaches of a broken marriage.

Special attention should also be given to the child or children. When children feel they have to take sides or are made to choose between the two parents, use **Scleranthus** to treat the confusion that comes by bringing the vacillating mind to balance and peace. The **Willow** child will resent the breakup and one or both parents. Unable to forgive, they can bear these grudges throughout their lives and create even more estrangement in the family.

Pine is necessary if the child feels guilty and responsible for the separation or the divorce, when they blame themselves for it. The flower essence releases the self-blame and guilt. A child draws all kinds of conclusions from every experience, which may be totally different from reality. Therefore communication is very important under such circumstances, to explain the truth clearly and to be fully honest and authentic with them. A 60-year-old man described how, at the age of nine, he was asked by his mother to make a choice between the life they had built for themselves or to go back to the father. On the airplane, his mother was crying and said she was going back to the father only because of him. The years to come were not happy ones, and so the little boy grew up bearing full responsibility for his mother's unhappiness and lived most of his life guilt ridden because of it. It was a very heavy burden to bear for one so young and truly an unnecessary one if the adults had the courage to take responsibility for their choices.

Sometimes the child finds that life stops there for them. Stuck in the memories of what it was like with both parents at one time, they miss out on much of their childhood. A 10-yr-old client, whose parents were separated, told me how much she always wanted them to come back together. She even described the curtains and rooms of the house the family once lived in. She became so absorbed in that desire, always ruminating over it that she could not be present to her surrounding, to school, and to the new way of life with her single mom. For this little girl, the essence **Honeysuckle** helped her to move on with her life.

● **Caregiving** – Some parents have to grapple with the unexpected – a child born with a life-threatening disease, autistic, deaf, physically or mentally handicapped. These children require a great deal of constant care, often into adulthood. The same situation could happen to children. A young woman described how at the age of ten, her mother was taken seriously ill and became bedridden. She had to grow up very quickly to run the household and take care of her siblings while her father was at work. Until today, she continues to be easily overwhelmed (**Elm**). Then there are adult children who have to care for the elderly parent stricken by illness or old age or dying. In all cases, the family not only has to deal with the grief but also make many sacrifices to accommodate the turn of events.

Here again **Star of Bethlehem** is useful for the initial grief and shock. **Walnut** can help everyone in the family make the necessary changes in lifestyle, routine and schedule. Caregivers who are **Centaury** types would tend to neglect their own needs and take even less care of themselves. The **Impatiens** person, who suffers from impatience, would have difficulty in this role. Their snappy, irritable and short-tempered manner with those under their care makes it an unpleasant experience for all. A **Vervain** mother of an autistic child, herself highly strung and hyperactive, explained how angry she felt all the time that this had happened to her little boy; an outrage that can be pacified by the Vervain essence. So much of her exhaustion came from her own tendency to overdo. The **Oak** type, stoic and brave, plods on against all odds. They have a strong sense of duty to those who are dependent on them and would not stop at all cost, except when their body breaks down and they can no longer carry on. The Oak essence helps to balance this tendency and relieve the frustration they feel when physically indisposed to carry on their responsibilities, thus allowing them to heal properly.

Other common essences indicated by long-term caregiving are **Olive** for exhaustion and **Elm** for feeling overwhelmed. Those caring for autistic children are highly stressed by their hyperactivity and unpredictability. **Rescue Remedy** can come to the rescue. One mother, who was advised to spray the Rescue Remedy on her child, found that it had a calming effect on him. Parents' nerves stretched to tethers can be restored by **Cherry Plum**. **Gorse** is indicated if every therapy is failing and feelings of helplessness and hopelessness prevail. Despite the best of intentions, undesired feelings of resentment can arise even for those under our care. **Willow** can wash away the bitterness of resentment.

The decision to put an elderly parent into a nursing home is probably one of the most difficult to make. If you feel torn and cannot decide on the best choice in the given situation, **Scleranthus** can help to bring the needed clarity and certainty. For some, the mere contemplation of such an option stirs up guilt for it is often seen as a lack of filial piety. Some readers may resent the suggestion that all a guilty person has to do is to take an essence regardless of whether the action is right or not. This is not how the **Pine** essence works. Actually, taking Pine helps to purify the mind of self-centered guilt and blame so the person can better assess the most beneficial course of action for all concerned.

• **Death and Dying** – Death is eventually unavoidable in every family, but death can also come prematurely and suddenly. A child lost at birth, another killed by an accident; a husband losing his life at his job or taken away by cancer, or an elderly parent who has come to the end of her life. **Star of Bethlehem** is the most important essence to deal with the inevitable shock and grief that accompanies such events. **Walnut** is helpful for the major transition and adjustment period that follows. It enables everyone to adapt to changes in lifestyle, family routine and the absence of a loved one.

Deep attachment between individuals can make the transition an emotionally difficult one. A young woman in her twenties lost her brother, whom she worshipped, to an air crash. Years later, she still cried over the loss of him. She thought of him often with great fondness, wishing and longing for his comforting presence. She depended on him a great deal while he was alive. After his death, she had difficulty knowing what to do and making decisions. As the years went by, she needed assurance in many areas of life and found herself having to consult others a great deal to come to a decision. **Star of Bethlehem** was given to clear the trauma and residual grief, **Honeysuckle**

to release attachment to the memories of her brother so she could move on with her life, and **Cerato** to help her trust her own judgment so she need not be unduly influenced and confused by others.

Death is the biggest transition we all have to make. We cannot stop anyone from dying when it is time for them to go, but we can help them to leave with peace and dignity. For the dying person, the essences can play an important role in facilitating their passing on. If the person is afraid of the dying process or death itself, **Mimulus** and **Aspen** can be explored; the former for the fear of death and the latter for fear of the unknown that comes after death. **Walnut** can help to stabilize the mind and cut off the influence of negative emotions of those they are leaving behind, **Star of Bethlehem** if the dying person is in much grief over the loss of life, of family, of everything familiar to them.

The way we live is the way we will die. Therefore we can help a **Willow** type to lay down the grudges they have borne so bitterly throughout their lives, and allow forgiveness to heal them and the people involved. We can use **Pine** to assuage the guilt of a parent who leaves behind young children to fend for themselves. We can help the **Vervain** angered by the injustice of the illness that afflicts them and the prospect of an unplanned death to reach some peace inside. **Honeysuckle** can help the individual who suffers from regrets over things they have or have not done in this life and are unable to let go. The essence releases attachment to these memories and allows them to move on peacefully.

There are of course many more challenges and issues faced by families. Each family is unique in its burden of these and it is therefore impossible to cover every one of them. Hopefully, the examples presented in this chapter have given readers a glimpse of how valuable the essences can be to reduce the problems in any family. More importantly, they are intended to make you aware that what we normally assume to be an unchangeable family reality can actually be transformed with the correct understanding and essences.

7

Growing Up as a Parent

Some working mothers who return to child-rearing after having built themselves a career would tell you that it is far more challenging to manage a household with kids than to work in the office. It is not because of the lack of monetary incentive, or position and power, but rather the daily task of being challenged as a human being. Facing a child everyday, their needs and their ways, is demanding. Interacting with another human being to such an intense degree constantly tests our beliefs, perceptions and our limitations. Most adults know that they can hardly hold a child fully responsible for their actions, yet despite their intention to love and provide the best care and nurturing, the best of mothers and fathers still experience times of despair, frustration, anger towards their children as well as moments of heartaches.

This chapter explores a sampling of parental types to help readers understand how such personality traits create stress and limitations in the parenting role and lead to unhealthy relationships with their offspring. The sampling is by no means exhaustive, but clearly demonstrates how many of the mental-emotional issues in parenting can be alleviated by the essences alone.

As we go through each type, it is important to remember that each trait can range from light passing states to long-term habitual patterns. We can all suffer from temporary states of such imbalances even if we are not of that type. The essential type has been more graphically described to bring the character alive, so you will have an easier time identifying essences for yourself or those you are helping. The purpose is also to demonstrate how each internal disharmony brings on the individual type of suffering. Each type can be in positive balance or in negative imbalance, but the essences are used here to denote the disharmonious states.

The Fearful Red Chestnut

The **Red Chestnut** parent is overly concerned about their children's welfare, health and safety. Concern for those we love is a natural response but in such a personality, it is rapidly blown out of proportion. The concern becomes fear that plagues the mind with worries and anticipating the worst of any event. This state is common in new mothers who have little or no experience in taking care of a child, and do not know the difference between an unhealthy fearful state and a healthy, balanced concern.

This is the parent who instantly bundles up the child in layers of blankets when there is a light breeze. The slightest sneeze and they are whipping up the thermometer to check the child's temperature. They fret and stress for the child sitting for an exam, or getting married. They cannot sleep a wink when their son has his first weekend away from home at a camp. Or a new mother who uses suppositories to make sure her infant has regular bowel movement. As one Red Chestnut parent described it: "I worry about my children when I am happy; I worry about them when I am not."

Stress for a Red Chestnut parent comes from fear. They spend a better part of their time attempting to protect their children from their own fears. Red Chestnut types are unable to enjoy the child because theirs is a relationship based on fear. This fear has its negative effects on the children. Children who grow up in this environment, where fear is hovering around everything they do, learn to fear quickly and become fearful of a lot of things. A fearful concern at its extreme can turn the child into a future hypochondriac or emotional invalid.

Q.L has a 6-yr-old son who was diagnosed with autism a couple of years ago. She was suffering from exhaustion, feeling overwhelmed and stressed just keeping up with her son's hyperactivity. In addition, he was constantly on her mind and worried her. Because he had not fully developed his language skills, she was worried that he could not take care of himself at school, that teachers or schoolmates would bully him; she worried what would become of him in the future. A combination of **Olive** (exhaustion), **Elm** (overwhelmed), **Rescue Remedy** (stress) and **Red Chestnut** were given to her. The Red Chestnut lifted the fears off her mind so she was better able to enjoy her son and share more light-hearted moments with him.

The Apologetic Pine

The **Pine** trait is commonly found in the working mother. Nowadays, few women are in the traditional role as full-time mothers and homemakers. Many are in the workforce, usually out of economic necessity and sometimes the lure of a career. Torn between their natural mothering instinct to care for their own children and economics or career, they suffer much from guilt. Knowing that they do not spend enough time with their children, they fault themselves for not being a good parent. Knowing that they are not giving all they can at work, they fault themselves for not performing well enough in their career.

Pine parents heap pressure on themselves in this way. The demands and standards they place on themselves are unreasonable and sometimes inhumanly high; as such they always see themselves falling short in their roles. In addition to the pressure, the running commentary in their mind focuses on the things they are not doing right or enough, for which they blame and reproach themselves. They blame themselves when the child is sick, for the child's grades and even popularity in school. With grown-up children, they may blame themselves for failing marriages, businesses or unexpected misfortunes. They claim responsibility too easily for things that have gone wrong, even when it has nothing to do with them. This stream of negative self-talk makes them feel really bad about themselves.

In illness, a Pine parent can feel apologetic about getting sick, as if the illness is an indication of a faulty nature. L.J., diagnosed with breast cancer, was trying to recover after a mastectomy. Instead, her Pine trait did not allow her to rest and recuperate in peace. She felt guilty for having all the time she had on her hands, for not making a living, for not taking care of the family. Constantly she looked for the next thing to do to ease those guilty feelings, becoming so busy she had no time to attend to her own healing.

Where the Pine has really fallen short is to attach to themselves too many imaginary faults and to be overly responsible for everyone and everything. The individual loses perspective of the criteria for assessing themselves. Since the standards they set are unrealistically high, they are constantly striving for unattainable goals and never quite making it. This creates a false reality of deficiency and imperfection, which explains why they strive so hard to be perfect and why there is no room for mistakes in their lives. The emotional reaction to fault and guilt is too much to bear. It takes days, weeks or even months for such a perfectionist to get over something they have done wrong. In severe cases, this state can paralyze a person into inaction.

The Pine essence helps to relieve this imbalance and loss of perspective. It allows the person to sit well with the imperfections of their human reality and to become more realistic in their self-assessment. Self-blame and reproach cease as they permit themselves to make mistakes, forgive themselves and move on.

The Yes Centaury

You can recognize a **Centaury** easily by their good and giving nature. They are generous with their time, effort and service. However, they suffer from a weak sense of self – who they are, what they want and their own purpose. They lose who they are by constantly attending to others' lives. Their needs are relegated to the lowest priority, they draw no boundaries with people, and often serve and give beyond their capacity.

In their eagerness to appease, the Centaury parent gives in easily to their children. Saying no is a near impossibility for some and so disciplining poses a great challenge. For them, it is an unpleasant task; they do not like to say no and displease since they believe this to be unkind. Even when they try, they are too weak to assert themselves and be heard or taken seriously. They are taken advantage by family members and in situations outside the family where they have to stand up for their children. We may find, in some cases, children who rule their parents with their wishes and demands. They climb over the heads of their elders and do whatever they want. They may even manipulate and become verbally abusive to a meek and mild Centaury father or mother. Such circumstances are unfortunate for the children too, for they grow up without a well-defined and healthy framework of appropriate and inappropriate behavior and will experience difficulty in adjusting as adults.

The underlying problem of a Centaury is a lack of wisdom in their kindness. They mistake pleasing others for love; they focus their acts of love on giving others what they want instead of discerning and doing what is really good for them. Because of their inability to draw boundaries, Centaury types serve others beyond their resources and physical capacity. The **Olive** essence is an appropriate companion when they have become exhausted physically, mentally and emotionally. Another state that commonly accompanies the Centaury trait is the **Willow** resentment. Since Centaurys have no inner strength to speak up and express their wishes and needs, they do not get the things they want and become resentful. Moreover, since they cannot say no, they succumb to others' pressure even when it is something they do not want to do. Over time, this pattern brings on a growing resentment, which the Willow essence can release.

The Totalitarian Vine

The **Vine** personality enjoys a certainty and clarity which makes it easy for them to know exactly what to do in a situation, and they are usually right. They are natural leaders; people you find in leadership roles or who are quick to step out to take charge of an emergency situation. They are assuring people to have around when we need help. In an unbalanced state, they are not so popular. They have been described as domineering, overbearing, authoritarian, dictatorial, inflexible, demanding and controlling.

The Vine is the lawmaker of the family, the one who sets down the rules for how things should be. At an extreme, the Vine parent runs the household with an iron rod, deciding what the children should study, what careers to adopt, who to marry, where and how to live. The Vine's word is law and often perceived as law because of the certainty with which they speak and the power of their personality. Opposition is not well entertained and therefore often not given.

This example is of a man who has done very well for himself in life, climbing up the ladder to the position of director in a big company. His Vine trait comes in very handy for his work, which requires leadership in his field. However, he does not stop being a director when he enters his home. He runs his family as he runs a company. The child has his role – to study and do well. The wife too has her duties clearly spelled out – she is to be a chef in the kitchen, the perfect hostess in the living room, an expert in homemaking, and the saint of a mother. On days, he would swipe his finger along the sink and question his wife: "What is this scum doing here?" or "Why are the flowers in the garden not blooming?" After all, it is her job.

At times, like anybody else, the Vine can be wrong. Then their certainty, once a virtue, becomes an obscuring factor that blinds them. Few can convince a Vine that he is wrong. They are more commonly in positions of giving instructions and directions than in receiving feedback and engaging in discussion.

The strength and power of the Vine character is overpowering for most people. This domination is especially harmful to young ones who are trying to express and develop into who they are. Most children take the path of least resistance, which is to crawl back into themselves and adopt a submissive Centaury stance to cope with a Vine environment. The other option is open conflict, which is unpleasant and even painful. If the Vine parent is overtly bullying, the child may develop a Mimulus type of fear.

We need not be out of balance to this extreme to use Vine. We should open our mind to using it whenever we find ourselves wanting the child to do things our way all the time. Each essence covers a whole spectrum of severity – light Vine state to heavy Vine tendencies – and it is good to be aware that at all levels, a little help would go a long way to rebalance our perspective and soften our mind to other's views and ways of doing things.

The Critical And Intolerant Beech

A **Beech** person has an unfortunate habit of seeing faults and flaws. It is as if she or he is walking around with glasses that can only see wrong. For some, this perception is pervasive and many things make them unhappy. For others, it could be more selective and applied to only one or a few individuals. In either case, the Beech finds it difficult to see the positive and good. They are critical, judgmental and intolerant of others' idiosyncrasies, habits or differences. These feelings can be verbally expressed or sometimes seething under the surface but still evident in their body language.

As a parent, this faulting is projected onto the child. One mother of a 9-year-old boy put it strongly, "I've reached a point where I simply cannot stand him. Everything about him irritates me – the way he walks, the way he talks, the way he eats." Or the child who comes home with "A's" from school, only to be questioned, "Where are the 100 marks?" Nothing the youngster does can please or satisfy the parent. This is a household scarce of praises and compliments.

You can imagine the harm done to a child who grows up in an environment where nothing about him or what he does is ever right. Daily doses of criticism, judgement and nit-picking, no matter how small, will erode the confidence and self-worth of any child. Beech parents often produce Pine children, who learn to fault themselves as their parents have faulted them while they were growing up. Youngsters can mistakenly absorb all these perceived imperfections as the truth of who they are. As adults, they frequently suffocate not only from the Pine trait, but also need Larch for feeling inadequate in themselves, and/or Crab Apple for the low self-esteem, shame and embarrassment that comes from believing there is something innately bad and wrong about them. Some carry this burden for life.

The Beech parent has to understand that picking on their children does not help them to improve and grow. Such cruelty can only inflict suffering; therefore can never be qualified as acts of loving concern and good nurturing. The Beech condition is their own suffering, not the responsibility of their children. Before they can help their children, they need to first treat this mistaken perception. When that pattern is released, they are returned to a more realistic and positive assessment and will be in a better position to help and support their children. In some cases, parents may find that using Beech on themselves is sufficient to eliminate the problem altogether.

⊛ The Smothering Chicory

Chicory is the smothering parent, full of love and action. They pour attention onto their children, fussing and doing a lot for them. They can be possessive and manipulative in their love; they like to be surrounded by those they care for and bask in their attention and affection. They are easily offended when they do not get what they want. These are the parents who are quick to pull the guilt trip: "After all I've done for you!"

In illness, this type thrives amidst plenty of fussing. Sometimes, consciously or unconsciously, they use their illness to manipulate the family to get what they want. It may seem a bit bizarre that there might be people who do not want to get well, but the Chicory's logic is that if they can have their wishes this way, the illness is a useful ally and therefore they see no need in giving it up so readily.

Chicory parents have a strong and powerful presence in their children's lives. They often feel they know what is best for them, and so become overly involved with every aspect of their lives. Their meddling can stunt a child's growth and development. Because they do so much for their children, the latter grow up feeling weak and helpless and highly dependent on others. The children only know power and strength in the parents but are deprived of the chance to experience their own. Such an interfering and unhealthy relationship leads to conflicts when the children grow up, start to think for themselves and want to lead separate lives. Chicory parents have a hard time when it is time for their offspring to leave the nest. Some Chicory mothers are known to follow their sons into their marriages and create friction in another household because they cannot let go.

One of my clients was in his late forties when he came to see me. For all his life, G.V. had lived with his mother, who was a strong Chicory. Whenever his mother wanted to move to another place, he had to quit his job and relocate. He brought girlfriends home but never got married because his mother liked none of them. He became completely submissive and devoted to his mother, who eventually became the only companion in his life. This man buried his misery in alcohol while his mother continued to cultivate the co-dependency by becoming the strong one to pick him up and carry him through this unhappy chapter of his life. This Chicory mother's possessiveness successfully retained her son by her side until the power of essence therapy and love for another finally took over.

In this case, the son was given **Agrimony** for denial of his own feelings and desires, **Centaury** for his subservient attitude, **Willow** for the buried resentment, and **Chicory** because he exhibited the same trait of possessiveness and need for the mother's attention and presence. He later went on to cultivate his own interests, a life and family of his own.

The Chicory essence loosens the apron string and enables parents to respect and honor their children's individuality. Their love and support becomes unconditional and balanced, not as a way to fulfill their own needs but truly to give the children they have brought into the world a real chance of living from their own essence.

⊛ The Resentful Willow

Some pregnancies are unplanned and untimely accidents. When the woman does not have the choice or is not ready for motherhood, she may blame the child for taking away her freedom or career prospects. The mother carries the pregnancy with resentment and begrudges the unborn child. The responsibilities of bringing a child into the world can also prove too much for young parents who have yet to stabilize their own lives. Financial responsibilities are heavy and one parent may have to take on an additional job to make ends meet. Household chores increase and spouses may fight between themselves on who gets to do what and how much. Childcare takes up time, energy and effort and the mother may have to quit employment to do this. Sleep has to be sacrificed to wake up in the wee hours of the morning to change diapers or to care for a sick child the entire night. Parenting is a 24-hour job that demands many personal sacrifices, especially when the children are young.

For the **Willow** personality, it is hard to rejoice in parenthood. They view these sacrifices as unfair and unfortunate, and become despondent with bitterness and resentment, which spill over into their relationship with their children whether desired or not. I have worked with a number of adults who were treated this way in the early part of their lives. Their parents made known to them that they did not really want them, and resented them as an unwelcome burden. This resentment, spoken or unspoken, can continue through the years. Children who are given such messages often grow up insecure, unloved and unwanted.

The Willow state is more common than we think. It is active whenever we feel ourselves victims of circumstances and begin to feel sorry for ourselves. When we want to blame others and circumstances for the difficulties we face, instead of acknowledging our contributions to the situation. In parenting, Willow is a good essence to reach for when feelings of resentment towards the effort and sacrifices so necessary to parenting overwhelm us.

The Impatient Impatiens

The **Impatiens** character tends to be quick in their thoughts, speech and actions. This individual is competent, efficient and bright, and has little patience with those who are not. Their general perception of the world is that it is too slow.

At home, the Impatiens parent is easily irritated and frustrated by any display of inefficiency in spouse and children, whether at chores or at play. Slowness is unforgivable. They become irritable, snappy and short-tempered when things are not up to speed. You will find them rushing everyone along, finishing sentences for them, precipitating actions for the family. In their impatience, the parent can take over dressing up the child, tying their shoelaces, doing their homework and continue to organize and complete tasks even for their grown-up children. Not only do they leave the children feeling rather slow, stupid and awkward, they also deprive them of the opportunities to learn to do things for themselves.

The Impatiens essence helps to relieve the inner tension of the individual. It is this mental and physical tension that drives them to such negative behavior. In balance, they are able to relax and be more present to spouse and children, enjoy them and accommodate their individual pace and timing in getting things done.

The Agrimony In Denial

Agrimony types have difficulty acknowledging, understanding and handling their inner experiences and emotions. They may be troubled, tormented, restless and worrying but do not know how to deal with these internal conflicts. They want peace internally and externally at all cost, and the price they are willing to pay is to keep up a pretense that all is well.

The Agrimony parent wears a jovial and happy face and they seldom let this guard down. Outside the family, they are often well-liked and make jolly good friends and company. They are the life of the party, the jokers and the clowns. There is always a smile on their face, even when the occasion does not warrant one. Unable to face their own emotions, they are quick to turn away and deny their children theirs. They make light of problems, their own and others'. It would be in line for an Agrimony parent to turn a blind eye to an anorexic daughter or a son with a drug addiction problem or even a spouse having an affair. The pattern is one of denial and suppression.

Their discomfort with truth and reality drives them to seek ways of distracting themselves. Some may turn to substances of abuse to numb and avoid their feelings, becoming alcoholics or drug addicts. They can also seek comfort in extra-marital affairs, or work, partying or food. When an Agrimony has an addiction, it is hard to help them because they are most likely to deny they have a problem. Little can be initiated to find a solution.

For this reason, this type is perhaps the most difficult to bring to therapy. If they are open to help, it will prove challenging to get them to face the issues and to be forthcoming about their emotions. Giving Agrimony is a good start to help the person ease their inner struggle and discomfort. As they reconnect with that which they have suppressed, they will find it easier to articulate their problems and receive the proper assistance. In severe cases, however, compassion may necessitate that we put together a formula based on our observation and knowledge of the person rather than on information given by them. A good dose of patience and understanding are also important ingredients for the healing process.

The Hurting Holly

Ever so often, we come across stories of parents who hurt and harm their children. The statistics in the US is quite alarming: In 1999, there was an estimated 826,000 victims of child maltreatment, nation-wide, and 1,100 were fatalities.[1] Research shows that of all children under age 5 murdered from 1976-2000, 31% were killed by fathers and 30% by mothers.[2] Every year, more than 200 women kill their children.[3] We may have read about newborns from unwanted pregnancies killed or abandoned in trashcans and alleyways. Some cultures commit infanticide and infant abandonment for economic reasons to this day. Child cruelty and injury are also reported in foster homes.

Here, we are not talking about the Cherry Plum type who impulsively and uncontrollably hit out at their children. The **Holly** who harms is not impulsive and out of control. They are fully conscious of their harmful intention and actions, and so cannot be excused on that score. Instead, they are blocked in their ability to love and suffer a distorted sensitivity to things or people that sets off the desire to hurt or harm. Their hearts are closed and cold.

You find this trait in the parent who consistently ill-treats their children, perhaps starving them, abusing them or chaining them up like prisoners in the house. We read of extreme cases in the papers or hear about them in the news: On August 8, 2001, Andrea Yates of Clear Lake, Texas, made the news headlines when she calmly and systematically drowned her five children in the bathtub. In another case, an 18-year-old arrived at her high-school prom, locked herself in a bathroom stall, gave birth to a boy and left him dead in a garbage can. She then touched herself up and returned to the dance floor.

In some cases, one child may be the object of abuse by the whole family. B.Z. was born retarded and the Holly type of ill-treatment started young for her. She was not allowed to sleep in the same quarters as the rest of the family, pinched, kicked, yelled at and beaten for no reason. At times, the angry parent or sibling would throw pails of water over her. The mere sight of her repulsed every member of the family and they hated her for what she was.

Fortunately, this is not a major disease amongst parents or children would have to suffer much. The public tends to view these parents as hopeless cases, mere criminals who deserve to be equally hated and punished.

Society contributes to the problem when it chooses to idealize women as the embodiment of universal motherly love, so that those who experience substantial emotional challenges in parenting have no place to voice their fears, impulses and concerns. Even such imbalances can be corrected with sufficient effective therapy.

Although most of us do not recognize the need for Holly, it is more prevalent in our lives than we would like to think. Whenever we feel mean, make a sarcastic remark to hurt someone, become suspicious or jealous, or intentionally sabotage another's effort, the Holly state is well and alive. You also see it in parents who, when exhausted, frustrated, angry and out of control with their emotions, find the mere sight of their child a hateful spectacle. The Holly essence can release the unwelcome oversensitivity and coldness of heart so we can recover our ability to love and care once again.

The Stoic Oak

Oak parents are a separate breed by themselves. Like the Oak tree, there is strength and bravery in the constitution of these individuals. They are dependable and responsible, steady as a rock. People love the Oak type because you can count on them any and all the time. Calm and collected, they do not fuss, complain or resent but carry out their life duties with a steady poise and perseverance that can only draw admiration and respect. Oak types therefore make a solid foundation for their children's lives – financially, emotionally and otherwise.

Behind the armor of stoic indestructibility lies an inability to heed the needs of their body and mind. Oak types never give up; they plod and struggle whatever the hardships. They endure and put up with a great deal. The only time when they stop dead in their tracks is when their body breaks down. Then they are annoyed and frustrated because they cannot get on with their work or duties. Because they are so reliable, more and more people depend on them over time. Seeing this makes it harder for the Oak to allow themselves to rest and recover properly.

An excellent example is a client in her thirties who owned and ran a health food store. She was feeling overworked but said, "Even if I'm tired, I'd still work." Once she was bedridden for two weeks from a bad allergy, medicated and hooked to an IV drip. She set up office by her bedside and continued to place the phone calls and pay the bills. She did not know how to put down her responsibilities and graciously accept the necessary rest.

This flower essence helps to relieve the despondency and frustration that comes when the Oak finds their strength and spirit waning. It teaches them to use their body and mind wisely, to provide the regular proper care and rest necessary to sustain joyous effort.

❀ The Apathetic Wild Rose

A *Wild Rose* parent suffers from apathy and resignation. They accept their lot in life and have no motivation to improve it. If they are in a dissatisfactory job, unhappy marriage or less than desired financial conditions, they make little effort to change this; they simply live with it. The Wild Rose is therefore unlikely to be a driven career person since they have little interest to make progress in their jobs. As such, they take no initiative to provide better living and financial conditions for their children. Poor grades and bad behavior are shrugged off as 'just the way they are'. They offer no encouragement, no guidance or discipline.

In public places, you can find a contented Wild Rose parent entertaining themselves while their children go rampant and disturb the peace. This parent type is not easily stirred to action. Gliding through life, they are passive and disinterested participants. They are not motivated to seek opportunities for their children, to help improve their school performance, or be troubled too much by their emotional problems. Their lackluster attitude brings a colorless, uninteresting and non-progressive quality to family life. Over time, they corner themselves into a rut. Wild Rose types often complain of low energy because they are blocked in their natural zest and liveliness.

The flower essence casts away the false perception that they have no choice but to accept what life delivers. It restores their enthusiasm and interest, and empowers them to action so they can expand and evolve as individuals and with the family as a whole. In this way, they also serve as better models for their children.

The Procrastinating Hornbeam

The **Hornbeam** parent may complain of being tired all the time but it is not a true fatigue. This type lacks energy because they are easily bored by daily routine and the chores of everyday living. This mental weariness makes them tired at the thought of doing them, and so they push them aside. It begins in the morning when they find it hard to get out of bed. They do not feel they have it in them to make it through the day. This is only a perception though, for once they start their engine going, they find that they are more than able to do the things they need to do. Of course, this delay in action can lead to many complications and is bound to affect child-rearing. Such parents are likely to put off parental responsibilities, guidance and effort.

Dysfunctional procrastination could lead to a messy household. One woman complained, "I have boxes blocking the corridor, stacks of dishes unwashed at the sink. I just don't have the energy to get to them." She was heavily overweight because she could not get on an exercise program. Her marriage was an abusive one but she had no energy to deal with that either. After taking Hornbeam, among other essences, she reported having more energy. She spent a whole day cleaning up her daughter's room with her, became more alert, organized and effective in taking care of things, arrived on time for appointments and prepared a whole school schedule for her girls for the new academic year.

The Hornbeam essence dispels the false notion of insufficient physical and emotional strength in these adults. The common feedback is that the time between thought and action is shortened significantly, and the person possesses greater energy that propels them to accomplish their goals, big and small. Daily life is no longer seen as a tiresome chore, but can be looked forward to with eagerness and enthusiasm.

❀ The Doubtful Cerato

The **Cerato** has a habit of invalidating and doubting their own wisdom and judgement. To compensate for this, they seek others' assurance to confirm that they have made the right choice. It takes forever to come to a decision and even after they have done so, doubts may still linger on, making it difficult to commit themselves wholly to their choice. This is how Cerato types make themselves vulnerable to the influences of others and, on unfortunate occasions, allow themselves to be led astray.

Parenting requires decision-making. A Cerato parent who faces constant difficulty with this can never be sure of the decisions they make for their children. A new mother who needs this essence will be uncertain of how to care for her infant. As the children grow older, she is unsure of the best way to bring up the children, how to discipline them, which school to send them to, what to do when they are sick or in need of help. She relies heavily on others' views and changes course with each advice given. The doubts and uncertainty that shrouds a Cerato parent makes an unhealthy and confusing environment for the children. They too have to change course with their parent's ever-changing mind.

This particular flower essence reconnects this type to their inner wisdom. It promotes faith in their judgment so they can proceed with certainty in their lives. It also helps them to understand that others' opinions and choices are not necessarily the right ones for them. Thus, they begin to learn how to empower themselves and to take charge of their own direction as well as that of their family.

❀ The Overwhelmed Elm

The feeling of being overwhelmed is common for parents. In the US, many single mothers work two to three jobs and juggle that with raising children. In the lower income bracket, both husband and wife may have to do the same to make ends meet. A working mother who has to prove herself in the professional arena and then go home to be a good mother can be stretched beyond her limits. Under such circumstances, even the most competent and most capable amongst us is going to feel overwhelmed.

When people do so much and for long stretches of time, their confidence crumbles under the weight of their load. When overwhelmed, a person goes into a state of doubt; they are not sure they can continue their responsibilities and begin to lose confidence in themselves. **Elm** is a useful essence to restore perspective and faith in their capacity and abilities. On top of using the essence, the Elm type needs to learn and respect their limitations for, so often, it is this blindness that causes them to overburden themselves.

❀ Significance of Parental Types

The understanding of essence types bears significant implications for parents. They can begin to understand how certain traits generate stress for them in the process of bringing up their children, how their particular sensitivities are triggered and why they respond the way they do. More importantly, they learn personal responsibility for their contributions to problems with their children. For those who feel they are failing badly as parents, this chapter will give them the hope that every issue is not fixed and hopeless. The case examples given demonstrate the opportunity within each challenge that exists to transform their parenting experience into an educational and pleasurable one. With the essences, they too can grow and evolve as their children grow and evolve.

---

[1]Fathers For Life, retrieved from http://www.fathersforlife.org/articles/report/resptojw.htm.
[2]Bureau of Justice Statistics, retrieved from http://www.s ojp.usdoj.gov/bjs/homicide/children.htm
[3]American Anthropological Association, retrieved from http//www.aaanet.org/press/motherskillingchildrenhtm.

Nurturing Your Child

"A small child has decided to paint the picture of a house in time for her mother's birthday. In her mind the house is already painted; she knows what is to be like down to the very smallest detail, there remains only to put it on paper.

The picture is finished in time for the birthday. To the very best of her ability she has put her idea of a house into form. It is a work of art because it is all her very own, every stroke done out of love for her mother, every window, every door painted in with the conviction that it is meant to be there. Even if it looks like a haystack, it is the most perfect house that has ever been painted: it is a success because the little artist has put her whole heart and soul, her whole being into the doing of it.

This is health, this is success and happiness and true service. Serving through love in perfect freedom in our own way.

So we come down into this world, knowing what picture we have to paint, having already mapped out our path through life, and all that remains for us to do is to put it into material form. We pass along full of joy and interest, concentrating all our attention upon the perfecting of that picture, and to the very best of our ability translating our own thoughts and aims into the physical life of whatever environment we have chosen.

Then, if we follow from start to finish our very own ideals, our very own desires with all the strength we possess, there is no failure, our life has been a tremendous success, a healthy and a happy one.

The same little story of the child-painter will illustrate how, if we allow them, the difficulties of life may interfere with the success and happiness and health, and deter us from our purpose.

The child is busily and happily painting when someone comes along and says: "why not put a window here, and a door there; and of course the garden path should go this way." The result in the child will be complete loss of interest in the work; she may go on: she may become cross, irritated, unhappy, afraid to refuse these suggestions; begin to hate the picture and perhaps tear it up: in fact, according to the type of child so will be the reaction.

The final picture may be a recognizable house, but it is an imperfect one and a failure because it is the interpretation of another's thoughts, not the child's. It is of no use as a birthday present because it may not be done in time, and the mother may have to wait another whole year for her gift.

This is disease, the re-action to interference. This is temporary failure and unhappiness: and this occurs when we allow others to interfere with our purpose in life and implant our minds doubt, or fear, or indifference."

Chapter 1, Free Thyself by Dr Edward Bach

❀ A Unique Essence

Individuality is a necessary ingredient to health and happiness and so much of success in life depends on following that which is unique to each of us – our innate nature. The human race is not made from a cookie-cutter assembly line. Every one of us knows that there is only one set of fingerprints or dental characteristics that belongs to us. The same is true of our entire mental and emotional constitution. We have our individual lessons to learn, areas to grow and expand, different sensitivities and vulnerabilities, and certain purposes to fulfill. We already carry the blueprint for our personal evolution when we enter this life.

Yet many of us fail to recognize this and instead spend most of life trying to fit into a mould; one not designed by us but by others who are merely drop-ins and passers-by on our path. They do not live our lives nor do we live theirs, yet we do not experience the autonomy to define our own success and happiness. So many grown-ups feel miserable about themselves, marrying incompatible mates, having a job they have no passion for, investing their life energy in things that bear little personal meaning and fulfillment. They exist and survive, some even well, but have never known what it is like to be joyously alive. Indeed, there are few who really know who they are, what they are about or stay true to their visions. Rather, they succumb to external pressure and interference and lose sight of themselves in the process of living.

This chapter is intended to provoke some soul-searching in parents. How much are you acknowledging and honoring that unique essence in your child? Are you willing and making efforts to protect that natural potential, nurture and grant it all the necessary conditions to grow and develop? What are you doing to clear the obstacles for your child's true expression and contribution? Or are you robbing your children of their individuality daily, trying too hard to make them just like you? Parenthood is, after all, not about the parents; it is about the child. Becoming an accomplished parent is to become aware of and to appreciate the differences in your child. It is celebrating them for who they are, not despoiling them by turning them into another you. What may have been good for you need not be appropriate for them.

For those parents who are daring and willing to take this different stance and perception of their role, the Bach system of essences is a wonderful and invaluable tool to achieve this. Here we will explore the challenges, obstacles and external interference that can threaten a child's individuality as he or she is growing up and, how as a parent, you can help to clear some of these hurdles with the essences.

Infants and Toddlers

Mothers with more than one child will tell you that each baby displays a unique character and traits from birth. As a rule, infants and toddlers do not conceal their emotions. Their behavior reflects their feelings and needs, and provides uncomplicated indications to the right essences. A happy, gurgling and smiling baby is an **Agrimony**; this type often exhibits a restlessness difficult to miss. **Chicory** is for the little one who clings, crying easily and needing much attention. This baby wants to be held and would have trouble weaning when it comes time to do so. The **Mimulus** baby is timid, frightened and easily startled. Some babies seem to be 'old souls' who live in a world of their own, taking no notice of anyone. They sleep a great deal and lack interest in feeding. These are the **Clematis** babies. You can spot a **Vervain** toddler from their high energy and activity level. They need to be doing a lot and can put up quite a bit of struggle. If you have a child who is taking an unusually long time in potty-training, speaking or walking, **Chestnut Bud** can be useful to clear the learning block. For the observant adult, it is therefore quite easy to put together a formula as needed.

Before I spoke to his mother, I-year-old Daniel had already gone through a ménage of diagnostic tests and surgery. Despite her skepticism, Sharon called after being referred by a friend who had earlier contacted me for help for her 3-year-old. The essences given to Daniel were **Agrimony** for his type, **Walnut** for his difficulty transitioning into feeding and sleeping, and **Crab Apple** to cleanse his system. His biological mother was a drug addict and he had tested positive for methamphetamine at birth; he also had residual medications in his system from previous treatment, tests and surgery. The ending of this story is this letter from his mother (Restoring the Face of a Baby). Three months after the initial phone consultation, Daniel and I met for the first time in Berkeley, and it was a delight to see his perfect cherubic face smiling into mine.

❀ Tackling Change

Change is prevalent from birth to adolescence to young adulthood, and **Walnut** is a must for every child because it facilitates the changes that come. The change in question could be of any kind: biological changes when the child is teething; hormonal changes in puberty; accompanying emotional changes

Restoring the Face of a Baby

Dear Soo Hwa,

Thank you so much for all your help with both our kids. I especially want to acknowledge the amazing results we have experienced with the Bach Flower Essences as you have recommended them for our son Daniel.

At 10 months, Daniel had a virus of some kind. Toward the end of the week, we noticed something 'funny' with his face. Well, long story short, as you know, after all the yucky tests the neurologist could come up to rule out certain things like meningitis, he was diagnosed with bilateral Bell's palsy. His face was partially paralyzed. They (the doctors) told us it would eventually go away. We didn't just want to wait and see. We pursued several alternative healing methods and didn't much care which one worked as long as Daniel's face went back to normal.

After contacting you and having a consultation, we started Daniel on the essences in every formula bottle all day. Your questions get right to the point and seem very intuitive. I really felt like you were getting to know Daniel over the phone and I trusted that you were putting together a safe combination that suited him. After 5 days, you told us to apply two of the doses each day topically. From that day forward, his face started coming back to normal. We kept up with that 'prescription' until the palsy was completely gone.

We are thrilled. And he is doing great. In fact, our 3-year-old is a great helper in remembering both Daniel's and her own 'fairy drops'.

Sincerely,

Sharon Krieger
Oakland, California

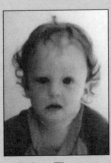
Before Therapy

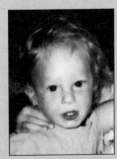
After Therapy

in adolescents, in the way they perceive themselves and the world, and their relationships with parents and the opposite sex. The external environment also changes. A young toddler beginning his school life has to adjust to the transition from the familiar confines of a family life to a strange environment – a school and classroom – with total strangers for teachers and classmates. From the perspective of the child, a quantum leap is required of him.

Some children experience extraordinary difficulties making this sudden shift from the small world they know to a huge and alien environment. When this happens, adults focus too much on their mission to get the child to school. Things can be more harmonious if we approach it a different way. Take a moment to put yourself in the little one's shoes, understand what is being asked of them and their difficulties in going through the process of change. This way, we arrive at a better perspective of why they are dragging their feet, dissolving into tears or rebelling and throwing temper tantrums whenever it is time to go to school. Instead of fighting their response, we can put our effort into better use by understanding the challenges they face and treating them accordingly. Help them through the transition by giving **Walnut, Mimulus** if there is fear, shyness, timidity, **Hornbeam** to give them that extra physical and emotional strength and energy to face the task, **Chicory** if they are clinging too much to mummy and daddy and cannot let them out of their sight. Sometimes they do not adjust well because they are holding onto the way life used to be. This is a **Honeysuckle** state; the essence cuts loose past attachments so they can move forward into the new chapter of their lives. The **Vervain** and **Vine** types can provide some turbulent resistance and opposition. These two essences will help elicit some co-operation. The parent too will benefit much from this exercise. Their wisdom and skill in tackling situations will improve as they begin to understand their child a little better each time.

The above difficulties do not only apply to young children. The move from secondary school to college and university is another leap. In primary and secondary schools, lessons are contained within a classroom. You know who you are sitting next to; you know who your teachers are. But in college or university, you find yourself sitting in a huge lecture hall, oftentimes beside strangers, with a lecturer you may never even have a chance to exchange words. It is another big transition and most of us do not appreciate the impact of such changes on us. A Walnut child would find it particularly difficult to adapt because of their hypersensitivity. They may take a much longer time to settle down, may struggle emotionally with adapting to a new crowd, new relationships and a new system, all of which may affect their studies. The physical stimuli in a new environment – the sights, the sounds, the smells, and the mass of people – also require some adjustments. Walnut keeps them balanced so that the inner upheaval caused by the outer changes can be minimized and they can function normally without too much disruption. **Honeysuckle** is a useful essence if they are stuck in the past, miserable from wishing and longing for the old and the familiar.

Food sensitivity can also trigger off negative emotions and behavior. A client described how his son, a normally pleasant boy, would scream and throw tantrums under the influence of chocolate. Studies have shown that there is too much sugar in the diet of children, and that certain allergies and behavioral problems can go away simply by eliminating these. The Walnut essence is an additional element to explore to help stabilize their physical and emotional systems.

Some children can be afraid of the uncertainty that change brings. L.I. was in her 20s when she came to see me. As a child, she found it difficult to sleep at night because she was afraid of the dark. The uppermost fear in her mind was that the boogie man would climb in through her bedroom window and get her. Often, she ran and hid under the blanket in her sister's bed. She lived with that fear all her life. It carried on as an underlying apprehension and anxiety ready to rear its ugly head, especially when there were impending big changes. Moving house was particularly tormenting for her. She would worry about the safety of the neighborhood and when she went out, she worried about rape and burglary. In this case, the essence **Aspen** quickly helped to put her at ease with the many unknowns that change brings.

Rescued by Bach Flower Essences

People from all over the world write to The Edward Bach Centre for help. The following story comes from Singapore, another case of a child who overcame her negative emotional-mental states and simultaneously healed from physical distress with the Bach Flower Essences.

*"A mother wrote for advice for her little daughter of 6 years old. Her condition was diagnosed as Juvenile Rheumatoid Arthritis brought on by emotional stress and fear of father who had had a severe accident and injury to his head, resulting in violent temper. The child had been ill for five weeks, with a temperature of 104, great pain in legs, back, hands and neck. The mother was advised to give her the **Rescue Remedy** for the seriousness of the condition, **Mimulus** for her fears and **Crab Apple** to cleanse the system. Gradually she responded, the temperature returning to normal, was much calmer and lost many of her fears, especially of the blood tests which formerly had made her hysterical and difficult to control. The last time, she sat down calmly and held out her arm which so amazed the pathologist that he said to her mother, "Have you been giving her some magical medicine?" She returned to school where she had always been considered a problem child. Now her teacher said she was happy and contented, a complete change of outlook, doing her work well."*

The Bach Remedy News Letter, Vol. 4 No. 19, Sept 1972
Published by Nora Weeks, The Edward Bach Centre, Mount Vernon.

Learning Difficulties

Chestnut Bud is good for slow learners, the children who make the same mistakes over and over again. In school, they lag behind in class because they take a much longer time to learn. Their more painful experience is to be labeled 'stupid' or 'dumb' by teachers or parents; having to wear this label damages their self-esteem and confidence for life. Such children also have difficulty breaking free of behavior patterns – biting fingernails, pinching another child, or other destructive behavior – and are socially difficult to train.

What is a Chestnut Bud's challenge? It is the inability to pay attention to the subjects that are being taught or the little lessons of life. This type has little retention or memory of what they have just experienced and slip easily into the same pattern over and over again. They are unable to learn well, build up skills and knowledge from their life experience and grow in wisdom over time. This trait, if left untreated, follows them into adulthood. As adults, they are unable to shake off harmful habits in relationship, lifestyle, or work. You find this, for example, in women who move from one abusive relationship to another. Some flower essence therapists have used this flower successfully to aid children with learning disabilities. It helps to eliminate that retention block and to experience a fuller learning potential.

One mother trying to help her daughter reported, "Before the essences, she had difficulty remembering what she had been taught. She also tends to retain the first input and even if it is wrong, she is not able to recall the corrected response. For example, when asked what majestic means, she described it as 'greeting the queen'. It was then explained to her that majestic means grand, related to grandeur. A day later when asked what majestic meant, she would respond 'greeting the queen'! After taking Chestnut Bud for three weeks, she seemed to retain and recall what she had learned better than before. This was reflected in her much improved grades." In fact, this youngster did so well she received an award for her improved school performance.

A **Larch** child suffers from an inferiority complex. They often compare themselves to others and view themselves as less than in every way and every situation. Their unhappiness springs from this mistaken self-perception and the accompanying experience of inadequacy and diffidence. When faced with a new challenge or opportunity, they expect to fail and do not even try. As one college boy said, "I don't want to play games with my classmates because I will lose anyway." When a Larch child grows up, she or he will continue to give up opportunities in careers and relationships, not taking the necessary risks to advance themselves or open their horizons. The Larch trait is their hurdle: "I cannot do it." "I am not going to accomplish it." "I am going to fail." When promotions come knocking on the door, they do not seize them and will never know what and how much they can really do and accomplish in their lifetime. The Larch essence ceases the endless stream of comparison, restores a balanced view and frees them of the need to use others as a standard for their performance.

Gentian is helpful to the child who becomes easily discouraged by difficulties in their studies. This is especially if they have studied hard and are still not getting the grades they want. As the disappointments build up, the child can lose heart and give up easily. This too can turn into a habitual response. When they grow up, they are unable to take the usual setbacks of life in stride. In relationship, at work or in the family, obstacles are blown out of proportion. They become downcast, may move into light depression and want to give up altogether. The flower essence helps to sustain the optimism and the faith to persevere. **Gorse**, for helplessness and hopelessness, is a great assistant when the Gentian has reached their endpoint.

In the United States alone, there are six million children medicated for behavioral problems. Ritalin and Adderral are the most popular medications for a basket of symptoms that are labeled Attention Deficit Disorder. Adults or children who suffer from this disorder are easily distracted, have difficulty staying focused on a task or paying attention, display disruptive behavior such as fidgeting, interrupting conversations, impulsive behavior and excessive physical activity. From the perspective of conventional medicine, these drugs are used to modify behavior by tinkering with brain function. According to the Bach system, we would explore the energetic imbalance and treat accordingly.

A **Clematis** child has difficulty with attention span because of a tendency to be lost in their thoughts. They are preoccupied with daydreams, imagination and fantasies. You see this in the child who can sit for hours staring into space, and who often feel drowsy and sleep a lot. Wrapped up in a world of their own, they have poor awareness of the environment and on goings around them. They pay little attention to what is taught in class or when spoken to. As a result, they can appear to be emotionally numb, clumsy, careless and even deficient.

Another personality type that lacks attention span is **Vervain**. This type of child holds and experiences tremendous surges of energy inside them. As the child attempts to rebalance him or herself, they engage in a stream of physical activities to use up the energy. They are hyperactive, bounce around because they cannot sit still in one place, and have to be exhausted to quieten down. For a child who has difficulty in a classroom sitting still to concentrate on their work because of their highly energetic nature and excessive bodily activity, Vervain helps them to unwind and relax and be more present.

An **Impatiens** child is quick and bright. They are quick in their thoughts, speech and actions, which have a rushed and hurried quality to them. They grasp things easily and are eager to move on, the reason why they are equally quick to lose interest and attention. They are readily irritable and frustrated by the pace in class, and have little patience for their classmates or teachers who are trying to explain the lessons to them. They do their homework hastily and often carelessly. This lack of ability to slow down to attend to and process information can result in an inability to learn properly. Physically they also move and fidget a lot in their eagerness to get on with the next thing they want to do. Waiting is not a favorite pastime of the Impatiens type. The flower essence helps to slow down their internal clock and relieves the physical and mental tension inside them. Patience is the opposing virtue of this essence type.

Boredom is a common phenomenon in the classroom. School children subjected to a routine easily lose interest in their work and surroundings. The mere thought of school and homework can cause them to mentally shut down, feel tired and put off doing what needs to be done. In this case, the child does not concentrate or hold his or her attention span because of a loss of enthusiasm for the lessons. **Hornbeam** is useful in such a case to lift the mental fatigue and lethargy that comes from boredom; it resuscitates interest and participation.

Just like some adults, the minds of some young people tend to latch onto passing thoughts. These thoughts circle repeatedly in their heads and they feel helpless to shake them off. Sometimes this **White Chestnut** trait can take the form of a fixation on certain objects or person or activity. One 18-year-old suffering from insomnia described it this way: "I cannot sleep at night. Stupid random things I see or feel during the day cannot be switched off at night. They keep going round in my head." This type of mental chatter also takes away their attention, making it difficult to concentrate on the task or learning at hand or to pay attention to conversations. It can result in mental exhaustion and congestion. The flower essence helps to relieve the mental chatter so they can have peace of mind and focus.

Sometimes you can find all these traits in a single individual. A 20-year-old university student complained of having problems sitting down and concentrating in class. Even when the lesson was interesting, her mind was elsewhere thinking about the errands to be done for the day. Her busy mind also made it hard for her to fall asleep at night (**White Chestnut**). She liked everything short and sweet and to the point, and became impatient when people try to explain things to her. This meant she often had to repeat her learning because she usually did not get the full picture the first time (**Impatiens**). Another reason she could not focus was her overconcern about the future. She had not finished her Bachelors degree but she was already planning her Masters (**Clematis**). She was anxious and apprehensive about the many unknowns in the future (**Aspen**). Since young, she had felt inferior, inadequate and used others as a standard for her performance (**Larch**). Everything was so tedious in her life, she had little interest or stimulation to stay on course and finish a task. Instead she kept putting them off (**Hornbeam**). This young woman had decided she was a slow learner and had brought much concern to her mother, who did not understand or know what to do with her. As you can see, these are simply personality traits that took her far away from her goals. After one treatment bottle, she reported feeling much better, less stressed in her studies and able to sleep again.

Social Interaction

The essences can also help to ease children into social interaction. Some children are extremely shy and timid. For them, social situations become painful experiences. They have a difficult time making friends and when they grow up into equally painfully shy adults, the challenge becomes more acute at work, where they have to interact with colleagues and business partners and in love relationships.

The **Mimulus** personality is afraid of people and the world at large. You see this type in the child who is shy, timid, blushes a great deal. They tend to move away from people rather than towards them. In front of strangers or a crowd, they become tongue-tied. Sometimes the fear is so strong that they stammer and stutter. The essence helps them to overcome that fear, and to open themselves up the world and to people. It provides them with the courage to embrace their lives and the world.

Children who spend a lot of time by themselves in childhood often develop the **Water Violet** trait. It could be that they were the only child, or the only girl or boy, or born into such a big family that they could not receive much attention from the parents. These children become habituated to their own company. They learn to play alone and to entertain themselves, and can suffer from loneliness and isolation. If the child does not outgrow this trait, he or she will find it increasingly difficult and awkward to interact socially. In some severe cases, children or adults become reclusive and withdraw from society. The loneliness and isolation intensify further, bringing on many types of illnesses. The flower essence dispels the sense of separateness from others, and puts them at ease with people. It also clears away the anguish of loneliness.

If a child is a bully at school, **Vine** should be explored. School bullies like to dominate other children, to impose their wishes and demand to be obeyed. **Holly** can also be used in combination if there is evidence of cold-hearted malice and sadism, and a delight in hurting others. **Beech** is applicable if the child is picking on those who are different, for example, children from a different race, religion, skin color, or who dress differently or speak differently. The Beech essence alleviates the suffering that comes from such intolerances. **Cherry Plum** will help if the child loses control easily and become verbally or physically abusive.

Centaury children are people-pleasers and therefore would be easily taken advantage of by others. School bullies can sense and will target Centaury types who are too weak to stand up for themselves. Such children often suffer in silence and the essence can give a boost to their self-worth and assertion. A **Vervain** or another Vine would not put up with bullying readily; they would fight back. These stronger personality types are common in school gangsters and leaders of such.

⚜ Teenage Years

Teenage years are a volatile and precarious period. At a time when teenagers are developing into individuals and discovering who they are, they are also the target of the mass media. Technology has turned the media into the most powerful and pervasive influence on young consumers today. Radio, television, magazines, movies, videos, advertising, the entertainment culture, and especially the internet all have a say in shaping and moulding your teenager's mind.

Daily by the minute, teenagers are exposed to all types of false ideals and made more image conscious than ever. The perfect body, the perfect look, the perfect and coolest thing to do, what they should wear, drink, do, how they should talk and act. There is even a website that teaches young girls how to turn anorexic to achieve the 'thin is beautiful' ideal. Added to this is the peer pressure to be accepted and be part of the trend of smoking cigarettes, taking drugs, drinking alcohol and having sex. There is tremendous exposure to all these influences and the impact on youngsters is profound and far-reaching.

The influence of the media is here to stay and parents are limited in their ability to control it or the environment to which their children are exposed. Teenagers, with little discriminating wisdom and plenty of desire to

A Gentle Process for Healing Your Life Once and for All!
by Melodie Pohorsky

I have been working to heal myself for many years and remove what felt like blocks to my effectiveness in life. I was battling depression, trying to set boundaries with the people in my life, healing past hurts from childhood and other issues that seemed to persist even with years of counseling, hypnotherapy, massage therapy, and even anti-depressants. I would notice improvements but still the feeling of being blocked in my life persisted. Finally, in what I believe was an answer to a prayer, I was introduced to Soo Hwa and the practices of Bach Flower Essences.

I began to incorporate taking the drops into my life very easily. I'd keep the bottle in a convenient place and would take four drops four times a day. Over time, I noticed subtle differences in myself. Situations that would normally upset me no longer caused me stress. It was easier for me to set boundaries with the people in my life. Over time, I was no longer struggling to get through each day but feeling a sense of well-being and energy that propelled me to accomplish my goals.

After I had experienced such positive results, I brought my 10-year-old daughter to Soo Hwa. Christine was experiencing spontaneous outbursts of anger and had put on some weight around her stomach. I felt that she had some emotional issues that were causing the physical symptoms. Our chiropractor had given her some supplements that seemed to help to a degree with her stomach but it had not completely healed. It was very easy to get her to take the drops on her own where it had been a struggle each day to get her to take the supplements which were in pill form. Over the next few weeks, as the drops performed their energetic magic on my daughter, she began to feel calmer and her stomach was healing. Now, her stomach is healed and she seldom has an outburst.

My teenage daughter benefited from the Bach Flower Essences as well. She witnessed the changes in her sister and was intrigued by the fact that she was actually beginning to enjoy her company! After two sessions with Soo Hwa, she began to take her own drops. She felt positive changes in her energy almost immediately. Being a teenager is a tough job and the essences helped her to feel more comfortable with herself.

I am very thankful to be led to the Bach Flower Essences. They have made such a difference in my life and yet are affordable, safe, non-invasive, and so subtly powerful. I highly recommend that anyone interested in living their life to the fullest and/or healing your emotional life give them a try.

be liked and accepted, are willing players in the media's game of persuasion. They can develop either way: constructive or destructive. Therefore it is very crucial during this stage of development to stabilize their inner state and to minimize the impact of the messages. The **Walnut** essence helps them to stay connected with their natural essence, so they can maintain an individuality and balance amidst the bombardment of the media. Walnut protects them from undesirable influences. **Cherry Plum** is also necessary when they feel they are going out of control, bending to pressure to smoke, take drugs or have sex. Driven by the impulse to conform, they fear losing control of themselves, knowing what they are going to do to be wrong and yet not able to contain themselves.

With the biological changes happening in their bodies, **Walnut** can be useful to facilitate the changes and **Scleranthus** to stabilize the mood swings. **Crab Apple** is very relevant to this age range because teenagers are highly self-conscious about their bodies. Too fat, too thin, too round, too flat, too short, too tall … there are many things to complain about when it comes to the body. The Crab Apple teen would be upset and obsessed with the mole on their face, acne, pimples or hairy legs. They suffer from shame and embarrassment, which can be cleansed by this essence. Anorexics and bulimics are often related to Crab Apple types; they latch onto some imaginary fault in their bodies and work extremely hard to correct it. Blinded by a negative perception of their body, they suffer much from an obsessive concern over it.

K.D. was a 14-yr-old boy who had become house bound. His mother came to the session on his behalf and described him as a very self-conscious child. He was scrawny, smaller and shorter than the other boys in school and was being bullied by some of them. He was easily upset if anyone made a comment about his hairdo, his clothes and how he looked. At some point, he decided on his own not to go back to school anymore. His mother believed that he had become consumed by his concern over his appearance and his fear of the bullies. He was given **Crab Apple** to cleanse his negative thoughts about his appearance, **Mimulus** for the fear of the bullies and his shyness from young, **Aspen** for his underlying anxiety and apprehension about school and **Centaury** for his easy-going yes-man attitude.

The **Hornbeam** and **Wild Rose** states are equally common among teenagers. The Hornbeam boredom and lack of interest in things routine lend themselves to laziness and procrastination. Wild Rose is for youngsters who lack initiative and make little effort to better themselves. Bland individuals who exhibit little joy, they simply allow life to happen to them. Parents who complain of children who 'cannot be bothered' to do a lot of things can use this flower essence to inject a dose of zest and liveliness into them.

Young Adults

The issues teenagers experience often follow them into young adulthood, especially when there has been no attempt made to deal with and resolve them. While they are allowed to be carefree in their younger days, as adults-to-be, they have to think ahead for their future and face responsibilities. Even if they are not concerned, they are pressured into being concerned. Depending on the personality traits, they respond to this pressure accordingly.

S.K. was a first year student at university. She had been seeing a psychologist for some time because she was no longer able to continue with her studies. She was suffering from an acute **Cherry Plum** state, losing control of herself everywhere. She spoke of breaking down into tears while standing in the canteen; getting up on a bus to go to campus and en route, jumping off and heading home when fear overran her mind. She threw temper tantrums at her parents, ate uncontrollably, could not sleep and had suicidal thoughts. These were signs of severe loss of control in every aspect of her life, for which Cherry Plum was indicated. **Rescue Remedy** was useful to alleviate the panic attacks. In session, it became obvious that she was pushing herself too hard to perform well (**Pine**) for the adults in her life and forcing herself to study things that she hated. **Walnut** was added to cut off the strong external influences.

Wild Oat is an essence of increasing importance as your child gets older. The Wild Oat dilemma relates to career, vocation or on a larger scale, one's direction and path in life. At some point, every one of us has to deal with this question. For young adults, it comes after schooling has been completed and one leaves college or university with a degree and a decision on how to use it. At a later period in life, in middle age, there often creeps into people the need to re-evaluate this decision and to initiate a new chapter and direction for themselves. Wild Oat is clearly useful in such mid-life issues as well.

This flower essence is indicated whenever we feel confused or blocked, not necessary in life, but also with specific problems and situations. The negative Wild Oat state is analogous to driving on a freeway without signage. Without the signs, we lose our bearing and become lost. Giving Wild Oat restores clarity and certainty to the mind by establishing a direction or pathway out of the confusion.

There are distinct Wild Oat types who are multi-talented individuals and who do well in everything they set their minds to do. However, unclear about their personal direction in life, they drift from one job to another, one career to another, one hobby to another, one relationship to another. Over time, they become frustrated because they are unable to find fulfillment and satisfaction in whatever they are doing, and feel that life is passing them by. Wild Oat grants them the ability to know what truly fulfills them and settle down. This essence is therefore useful in vocational and career counseling, and can help to eliminate years of searching and frustration.

Even if your child has no obvious challenges facing them, it is wise to become aware of their tendencies and sensitivities. Under stress, their personality traits become unexpectedly pronounced and may be a sign of impending illness. A Clematis child becomes more sleepy and drowsy; a Mimulus child more fearful and a Chicory child turns clingy and needy. You can use the appropriate essences to quickly aid them to balance and therefore to health.

Learning about the essences is also a way for parents to better understand their children, which in turns makes parental guidance and aid flow more easily. The conflicts, judgments, fears and melodrama can be minimized for a more harmonious family environment. This can save the child years of suffering, and for the parents, years of trying to fix them when they are older.

Part IV

Conclusion

| To gain freedom, give freedom. | Dr Edward Bach Free Thyself |

9
Making Conscious Choices

Growth involves developing a higher degree of self-awareness and volition in the decisions we make in life. Therefore, even as you use the essences to relieve yourself and your children from undesired traits and habits, you must also become increasingly intentional in how and where you are taking everyone in the process of parenting. Are you going to emerge more matured, patient and giving from the office of parenthood or are you going to turn picky, grumpy and controlling? Has your child been encouraged to think and act for themselves and taught independence, individuality and freedom or have they learned, during their time with you, to comply, to hold their tongues, to suppress themselves and to become responsible for your faults and unhappiness?

These are serious questions every parent should ask of themselves before even considering the conception of a child. Most couples bring little awareness into their roles as parents. They have children because that is the expected thing to do after marriage. They bring up their children the only way they know – usually the way they were brought up – or swing to the other extreme of doing everything opposite to how they were brought up. Perhaps the one consistent change is that most parents are able to provide greater physical comfort and resources to their children than they were able to enjoy when young. These material things, however, do not mould the children. It is the interpersonal dynamics with adults of influence that craft the child's personality.

Past generations of women produce babies because it was their wifely duty; nobody asked them if they wanted to have children or not. We would think that as people become more literate and educated over time, they would make wiser choices. Educated couples still have the most archaic reasons for having children. Asian men who want a son to carry on the bloodline will continue to breed till they get one. Tremendous effort and resources are invested into the fusion of an egg and sperm destined to carry on the family name. Working women continue to perform their wifely function unquestioningly, and many couples see children as a means to fulfill and complete themselves or raise them as a form of insurance for old age – someone to care and provide for them when they get old. One professional woman spent years of effort in a fertility clinic to conceive just to prove her fertility to her in-laws and then wonder and fret that her child is not close to her. She had never wanted her in the first place anyway. Then there are many young people who wantonly and carelessly give in to their sexual impulses and, along the way, produce little 'accidents' that they never wanted and therefore abandon.

The office of parenthood is a privilege that ought not to be taken so lightly. A child is not a commodity to be brought into the world to serve your cause and your needs. It is another life, precious to be respected and honored in its own right. Therefore, the clearer you are about why you need or want a child and how you want to bring it up, the clearer your path in parenting will be. Otherwise, unconscious desires can turn into a complicated nightmare and unconscious behavior as a parent turn into unconscious habits and beliefs that are passed down from one generation to another, with no hope of breaking the cycle.

In his book *Heal Thyself*, Dr Bach dedicated an entire chapter on the importance of cultivating individuality as an essential step on the path to true health. For this purpose, he gave serious treatment to the subject of parenthood. Before we close this book together, I too would like to leave you with a few parting thoughts on this subject.

> • *Your child is an independent being who has his or her own path of evolution and purpose in life. He or she is not an extension of who you are. So, at all times, give them the freedom to be different from you.*

Too many tragedies have happened when people try to interfere with, manipulate and control the destinies of another. The public cries out against the tyranny of dictators and how they use their citizens; but such tyranny exists also in the household where it goes on silent and unnoticed. The slow killing of the individual spirit happens daily by the minute with each oppression, rejection, ridicule and criticism. Parents may feel that they have the right to do this, by virtue of bringing the child into this world and having to make the sacrifices to care and protect it. They feel that they own the child, but Dr Bach would not have agreed with such a sentiment more.

In Chapter V of his book *Heal Thyself,* he stated: "Parenthood is a sacred duty … It carries with it nothing but service and calls for no obligation in return from the young …" He went on to say, "Parents should be particularly on guard against any desire to mould the young personality according to their own ideas or wishes, and should refrain from any undue control or demand of favors in return for their natural duty and divine privilege of being the means of helping a soul to contact the world. Any desire for control, or wish to shape the young life for personal motives, is a terrible form of greed and should never be countenanced, for if in the young father or mother this takes root it will in later years lead them to be veritable vampires. If there is the least desire to dominate, it should be checked at the onset. We must refuse to be under the slavery of greed, which compels in us the wish to possess others. We must encourage in ourselves the art of giving, and develop this until it has washed out by its sacrifice every trace of adverse action."

For those parents who are expecting a share of their children's life, Dr Bach warned of the potential tragedy in his writing *Free Thyself:* "So many suppress their real desires and become square pegs in round holes: through the wishes of a parent a son may become a solicitor, a soldier, a business man, when his true desire is to become a carpenter; or through the ambitions of a mother to see her daughter well married, the world may lose another Florence Nightingale. This sense of duty is then a false sense of duty, and a disservice to the world; it results in unhappiness and, probably, the greater part of a lifetime wasted before the mistake can be rectified."

Too many have died without ever knowing who they are, or doing what they have always wanted to do. Why do you think so many people feel they live empty lives? Not because they are empty individuals without dreams and with nothing to contribute to the world, but because they have been used by more dominant personalities, or crossed in their paths by interfering ones. Because they are too weak, too distracted, too afraid to follow when their dreams call. Life-long wishes harbor silently in their hearts as they pursue the business of living, not knowing that only when that spark within is lighted is there really life for them. The famous mid-life crisis is easy to understand in this light. The majority spend the first half of their lives following the rules laid down by others. In the second half, some may wake up to themselves in the nick of time; others find it near impossible to reconnect and end up lost and confused for the remainder of their lives.

> • *When raising a child, adopt the view of perfection. Start with the premise that their true nature is pure, and then ask yourself: What difficulty is the child facing in expressing his or her essence? What can I do to clear away these obstacles so the beauty and perfection of that inner nature can shine through?*

There is nothing innately wrong with any child or any individual. We are all fundamentally whole; our true nature is pure and uncontaminated by the vibrations of our negative mental and emotional habits. Just like the mirror is unstained by its reflections or the sky by the clouds. We do, however, experience rather unique problems in expressing that essential nature. In flower essence therapy, we are not trying to fix, correct, or even balance a nature that is already whole. Rather we are treating to clear away the blocks to true expression. This is where I begin my work with clients. As a practitioner, I do not view a client as a bad or difficult person, no matter what issues they bring into the session or whatever shameful and shocking things they have done. My work is to help them refocus on the goodness and empower that, using the essences to release obstacles along the way.

If you too orientate your mind in this way, you will arrive at a totally new understanding of parenting. With this new wisdom, compassion and service arise spontaneously. Parenting need no longer be a tiresome burden or grudging obligation. It is an act of love to empower another individual to be all they can be and to give all they can give to the world. Many of today's social problems come about because there are too many bored, aimless, lost and unhappy people. Allow children to live themselves to the fullest and you will have a society of physically and emotionally sound individuals. All it takes is simply to adjust your view and the actions will follow.

> • *Your role as a parent is a sacred one of protecting and caring for that spark within your child that is unique to him or her, to provide all the necessary conditions for it to grow in strength and develop fully. Just as plants need sunlight and water, so does the potential of the child need love, encouragement and support to bear fruit.*

Parents, as guardians of the newcomer, are to provide all the necessary ingredients for success of this new life. To the best of their ability, to become a storehouse of spiritual, mental and physical guidance and resources for their children and at every stage of the journey, to offer every possible freedom for their unhampered development. They have to tend to their young ones the same way farmers tend to their crops.

Farmers who do not till the soil before seeding, and do not fertilize or water them, cannot even see the light of a seedling. Farmers who do not leave the seedlings alone once they start growing, but keep pulling them out to see how they are doing, kill the young plants prematurely. Those who abandon and neglect their crops are unlikely to see a harvest. Every stage has to be cultivated with attention and care. The same can be said for a human being who arrives into this world.

> • *Choose your battles wisely. Save them for the really important things, and do not waste them on trivia that leave only painful memories and bitter regrets.*

Many conflicts between parents and children come about because the adults have not laid out clear priorities in their parenting scheme. If you are the parent who picks on the child for how he eats, how she treats the living room sofa, what time he showers, think again about your priorities. Is your child more important or the family sofa? Is the negativity you leave on his or her mind more important or having your way all the time? Is your frustration and lack of fulfillment with your own life the fault of your child?

Think deeply about the consequences of your actions and minimize damage to your child as much as possible. Focus on the essential – those things that bring you and your child closer, that help you and your child to see the good and positive, that brings more laughter, love and joy into the relationship, more thoughtfulness and kindness in thoughts, speech and actions. We cannot 'fight evil with evil', only by bringing light and goodness back into our lives.

> • *See your children as your teacher. They are like mirrors held to your face everyday, showing you your habitual tendencies and unresolved issues, dark areas of stunted growth where you need work. They offer you a chance to learn, grow and mature with them.*

Without your children pressing your buttons, there is no anger, no sadness, no indignation, no resentment and also no opportunity to do something about them. Your children provide the safest environment for you to practice breaking free from old negative habits. They are also the most forgiving and most loving training partners. No matter how many times you fail, they still love you unconditionally.

You can choose to focus on this most precious opportunity to transform and mature yourself. As your child is growing up, you are also growing up and this can bond into a very beautiful relationship. Or you can choose to bypass this lesson and continue in the same habitual and mistaken perception: It is the child who irritates me, who is at fault, who is stupid or slow, who loses control, who is stubborn, who is strong-willed. Focusing in this way is an exercise that breeds and guarantees negativity between you and your child, unhappiness in your mind, and greater ignorance. Watch how your being respond to each option and based on your observation, take the choice that brings you greater inner peace and freedom.

I hope that your passage through this book has been both useful and enjoyable, and encourage you to explore Dr Bach's system of essences for yourself. Beliefs come and go; they change depending on the popular view of the times, or the popularity of the person presenting the view. They are as changeable as fashion. But no one can take away our experiences, which goes to show that the best way to know if something has truth or not is to test it ourselves. To do this with the Bach system, it means taking the essences.

There are many who swear by them because of their personal experiences. Nothing said against the essences can take away their faith and conviction. Then, of course, there are others who are waiting for proof before they will take action. In the meantime, they continue to suffer needlessly. If you check carefully, you will see a certain foolishness in this. Such people have given away their power to ascertain the truth for themselves. Instead they rely completely on others to tell them what is real and what is not, what is good for them and what is not. Consequently, they deprive themselves of healing for the sake of an opinion.

This unfortunate situation need not be if we know how to truly care for ourselves. We must not take our attitudes and habitual behavior for granted; nor should we rely completely upon them to see us through life. Each challenge thrown in our direction is a call to check and adjust our attitude and behavior, a call to re-examine assumptions and beliefs, a call to evolve and transcend old ways. When birds are in flight, they glide but make minor adjustments with the wings to keep them in the air. Similarly, to soar as human beings, we need to keep ourselves poised in a state of equilibrium by constantly tweaking and fine-tuning our perceptions, beliefs, and emotional states and bringing them closer to the truth of reality. Then, and only then, can we be assured of a safe and enjoyable flight through life.

End

Appendix

Let us remember that disease is a common enemy, and that every one of us who conquers a fragment of it is thereby helping not only himself but the whole of humanity.

Dr Edward Bach
Heal Thyself

Bibliography

Philosophy and History

⊛ Heal Thyself: An explanation of the real cause and cure of disease – Dr Edward Bach

⊛ The Medical Discoveries of Edward Bach Physician – Nora Weeks

⊛ The Original Writings of Edward Bach – Judy Howard & John Ramsell

⊛ The Story of Mount Vernon – Judy Howard

General Information on Bach Essences

⊛ Bach Flower Remedies: Questions & Answers – John Ramsell

⊛ Bach Flower Remedies Step by Step: A complete guide to selecting and using essences – Judy Howard

⊛ Bach Flower Therapy: Theory and Practice – Mechthild Scheffer

⊛ Illustrated Handbook of the Bach Flower Remedies – Philip M. Chancellor

⊛ The Bach Flower Remedies: Illustrations and Preparations – Nora Weeks & Victor Bullen

⊛ The Bach Remedies Repertory – F.J. Wheeler, M.D.

⊛ The Encyclopaedia of Bach Flower Therapy – Mechthild Scheffer

⊛ The Twelve Healers & Other Remedies – Dr Edward Bach

Specific Uses of Essences

⊛ Bach Flower Remedies for Men – Stefan Ball

⊛ Bach Flower Remedies for Women – Judy Howard

⊛ Bach Flower Remedies to the Rescue – Gregory Vlamis

⊛ Growing Up with Bach Flower Remedies: A guide to the use of remedies during childhood and adolescence – Judy Howard

Useful Contacts

The Dr Edward Bach Centre
Mount Vernon, Bakers Lane
Sotwell, Oxon
OX10 0PZ
United Kingdom
Tel: 44-14-9183-4678
Fax: 44-14-9182-5022
centre@bachcentre.com
www.bachcentre.com
International register of practitioners

Nelsonbach UK
Broadheath House
83 Parkside, Wimbledon
London SW19 5LP
United Kingdom
Tel: 44-20-8780-4200
Fax: 44-20-8780-5871
info@nelsonbach.com
www.bachfloweressences.co.uk
Worldwide distributors & training

Nelsonbach USA
100 Research Dr
Wilmington
MA 01887, USA
Sales: 1-800-319-9151
Education: 1-800-334-0843
Fax: 1-978-988-0233
info@nelsonbach.com
www.nelsonbach.com

Distributors in Asia & Australia

Living Commercial Ltd
48 A&C, Hamilton Comm. Bldg
558-560 Nathan Road
Kowloon, Hong Kong
Tel: 852-2625-4619
Fax: 852-2384-2333
bill@livingcomm.com

⊛

Purnama International Co. Ltd
Jingumae 4-24-23-101
Shibuya-ku,
Tokyo 150-001, Japan
Tel: 81-3-5411-7872
Fax: 81-3-5411-7874
master@purnama-intl.co.jp

⊛

Tree of Life Natural Remedies Sdn Bhd
Suite 3.10, Level 3
Menara Duta 2, Jalan 1/38B
Off Jalan Segambut
51200 Kuala Lumpur
Malaysia
Tel: 603-6250-2399
Fax: 603-6250-6399
suesie@treeofliferemedies.com

⊛

Essential Living (S) Pte Ltd
18B Carpenter Street
Singapore 059907
Tel: 65-6276-1380
Fax: 65-6276-1370
essliv@pacific.net.sg

Tech Join Taiwan Co. Ltd
8F-3, No.2, Section 2
Kingsan South Road
Taipei, Taiwan 106
Tel: 886-2-2397-95168
Fax: 886-2-2397-9519
techjoin@ms8.hinet.net

❈

Martin & Pleasance Pty Ltd
123 Dover Street
(PO Box 2054)
Richmond, Vic 3121
Australia
Tel: 61-39427-7422

In honor of the master healer
who resides in every being as
the potential to awaken
to original wholeness.

Soo Hwa

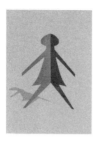

About the Author

Soo Hwa is a trained pharmacist with a research background in pharmaceutical chemistry and pharmacology. In USA, she pursued her interest in the healing arts to become a Bach® Foundation Registered Practitioner and an assessor, practitioner-teacher and mentor with the Bach® International Education Program. She is also a Certified Quantum-Touch® Practitioner and founded The SomEsse® Method, an approach unique to her practice.

Like Dr Bach, the foundation of her healing philosophy is that true health is only possible when individuals are empowered to live from their essence. SomEsse, which teaches the pathway from body to essence, applies this single understanding and explanation to multiple modalities to effect rapid and profound healing and growth in self-wisdom that makes healing complete.

Currently resident in USA, Soo Hwa teaches and consults in California, and periodically in Asia.

*I hope you have enjoyed this book and invite you
to share your experiences with the Bach Flower
Essences. Write to 1220-152 Tasman Dr, Sunnyvale,
CA 94089, USA, or send an email to Soo Hwa at
essences@softhome.net. I would love to hear
your stories and successes.*